# THE BHAGAVAD GITA WISDOM FOR YOUNG MINDS

## A LITTLE SEEKERS GUIDE

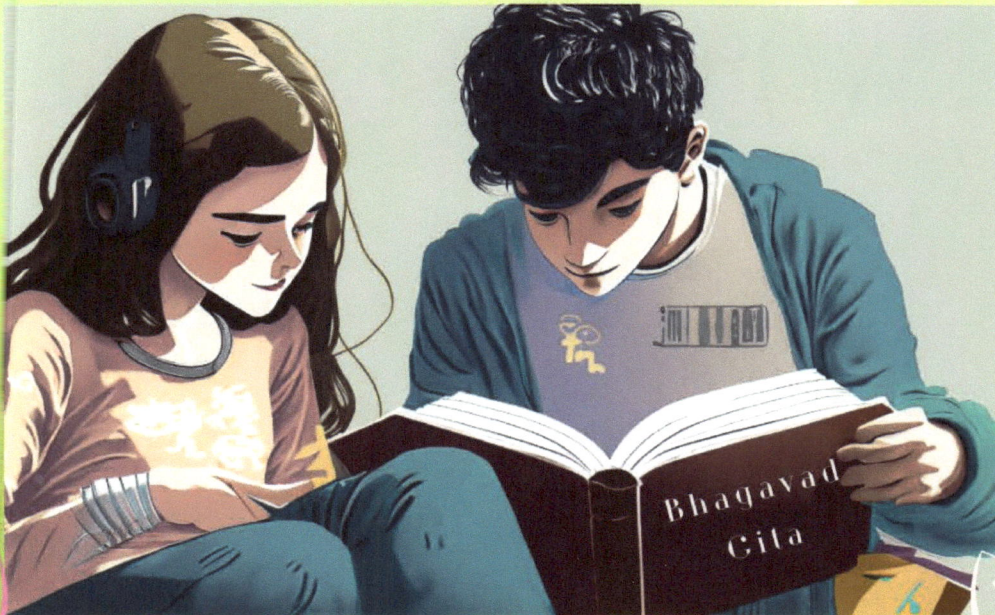

*"Big lessons, for little heroes!"*

## BY SUSHIL KHADKA

# The Bhagavad Gita Wisdom for Young Minds

## A Little Seekers Guide

*"Big lessons, for little heroes!"*

**SUSHIL KHADKA**

## Disclaimer

### Content and Interpretation:

The Bhagavad-Gita is a complex and multifaceted text with interpretations that have evolved over centuries. This book presents a simplified and youth-oriented understanding of the Gita's core themes. While we have strived for accuracy, it is not a substitute for in-depth study of the original text or guidance from qualified teachers.

We recommend consulting the following resources for further exploration:

- **The Bhagavad-Gita** For Children and Beginners by Ramananda Prasad, Ph.D.

- **The Bhagavad Gita As It Is** by A. C. Bhakti Vedanta Swami Prabhupada

### Accuracy and Errors:

Every effort has been made to ensure the accuracy of the information presented in this book. However, errors and omissions may exist. The publisher and authors disclaim any liability for damages arising from the use of the information contained herein.

### Copyright and Trademarks:

### Respect for All Faiths:

This book is intended to be a gentle introduction to the Bhagavad-Gita's wisdom and is presented with respect for all faiths and belief systems.

## Contents

# Preface

## Unveiling the Wisdom of the Bhagavad Gita for Young Minds

Forget dusty textbooks and cryptic Sanskrit verses! This book takes you on a thrilling adventure to unlock the timeless wisdom of the Bhagavad-Gita, specifically designed for young minds like yours.

Imagine the Gita as a hidden treasure map, leading you to the secrets revealed in the epic dialogue between Arjuna and Krishna. Here, the story unfolds in a captivating narrative that speaks directly to your experiences and challenges.

Think of this journey as best taken with a trusted guide – a teacher, parent, or mentor familiar with the Gita's teachings. Before we embark, let's set the scene. The legendary Kurukshetra war serves as a powerful metaphor for the internal battles we all face. The Bhagavad-Gita equips you with the tools to fight these battles with courage, integrity, and unwavering moral compass.

### Unleash Your Inner Explorer: Interactive Learning

This book isn't meant for passive reading; it's an interactive treasure hunt! Here are some ways to make the most of your adventure:

- **Chapter Quest:** Each chapter kicks off with a captivating introduction, unveiling key themes and igniting your curiosity. It's your mission to embark on this quest and discover the hidden gems within.

- **Student Spotlight:** Unleash your creativity! Think beyond the page and present the chapter's teachings in unique ways. Craft skits, debates, or even musical interpretations to share your understanding and spark lively discussions with your classmates.

- **Real-World Challenge:** Bridge the gap between ancient wisdom and your present-day life. Use relatable scenarios or role-playing exercises to see how the Gita's lessons play out in the modern world. This helps you apply these principles to your own experiences and become a moral compass for yourself and others.

## The Enduring Echo: Timeless Wisdom for Today

The Bhagavad-Gita isn't a relic of the past gathering dust on a shelf. It's a vibrant guide, offering timeless wisdom for navigating the complexities of life, no matter the era. It speaks of facing challenges head-on, staying true to your values, and leading a life of purpose – principles that resonate across generations.

Though the battles fought on the battlefield of Kurukshetra may seem far removed from our daily lives, the core message remains: the Gita equips us with the tools we need to stand tall amidst adversity, acting with integrity and moral clarity.

## Why Now, Why You?

In a world obsessed with constant progress and external validation, life can feel increasingly confusing. The Bhagavad-Gita offers a compass, reminding you of essential values that may get lost in the shuffle.

Young people today are bombarded with conflicting messages and pressured to conform to external expectations. This book empowers you to make conscious choices, navigate your world with a strong moral compass, and forge your own path.

The media often portrays success as a destination reached by any means necessary. The Gita, however, teaches us that true success is inextricably linked to ethical conduct. It emphasizes the importance of the journey as much as the destination.

## Weaving the Fabric of Humanity: The Importance of Dharma

The Bhagavad-Gita places great emphasis on Dharma, righteous conduct. It's more than just following social norms; it's the foundation for living a good life and building a thriving society. It's the very fabric that binds us together and creates a harmonious world.

Morality isn't a choice; it's an inherent part of who you are. As Swami Vivekananda eloquently stated, "How can you be a cheat or inhuman?" Dharma is the expression of your truest self.

## A Universal Invitation: Embark on Your Journey

The thirst for knowledge and meaning exists everywhere, regardless of wealth or circumstance. The Bhagavad-Gita offers nourishment for all. Reaching young minds is crucial to building a world that reflects our highest ideals.

This book is your invitation to embark on a journey of self-discovery, guided by the wisdom of the Bhagavad-Gita. Let's begin your adventure!

This revision focuses on the interactive and engaging nature of the book, emphasizing the "young explorer" theme. It also avoids specific references to other potentially plagiarized sources.

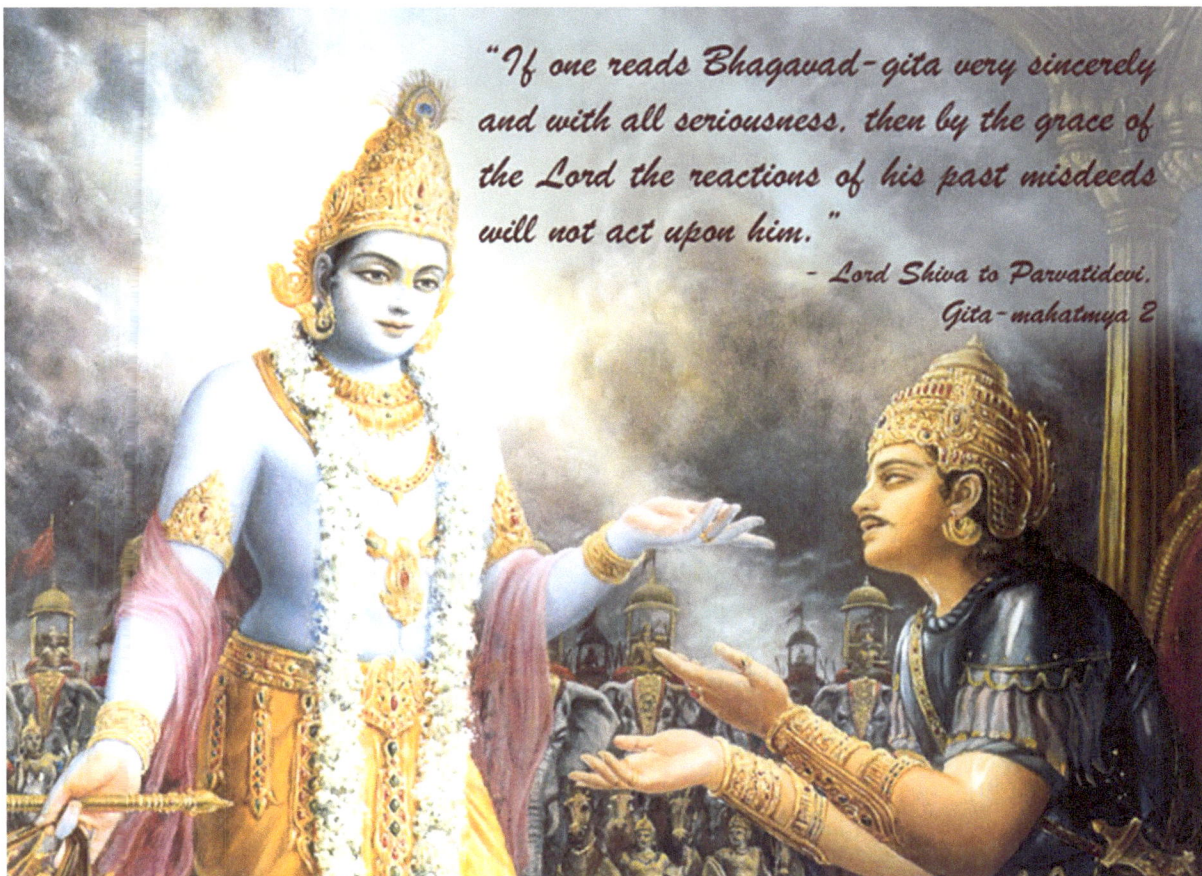

"If one reads Bhagavad-gita very sincerely and with all seriousness, then by the grace of the Lord the reactions of his past misdeeds will not act upon him."

— Lord Shiva to Parvatidevi. Gita-mahatmya 2

# Dedication

To the Kind Hearts Who Shine Brightest:

This book is dedicated to:

- **Lord Krishna, the ultimate teacher**: May his wisdom guide us on the path of selfless action and inner peace.

- **His Divine Grace A.C. Bhakti Vedanta Swami Srila Prabhupada**: Through his tireless efforts, the Bhagavad-Gita's wisdom becomes accessible for all.

- **My revered gurus and Param gurus**: Their guidance lights my way on the spiritual journey.

- **My parents**: Their love and support are the foundation for everything I do.

May all the curious minds and compassionate spirits who embark on adventures every day find joy in discovery, strength in selflessness, and the light that shines from within. Remember, even the smallest acts of kindness can ripple outward, making the world a brighter place.

With love and hope,

SUSHIL KHADKA

# Introduction

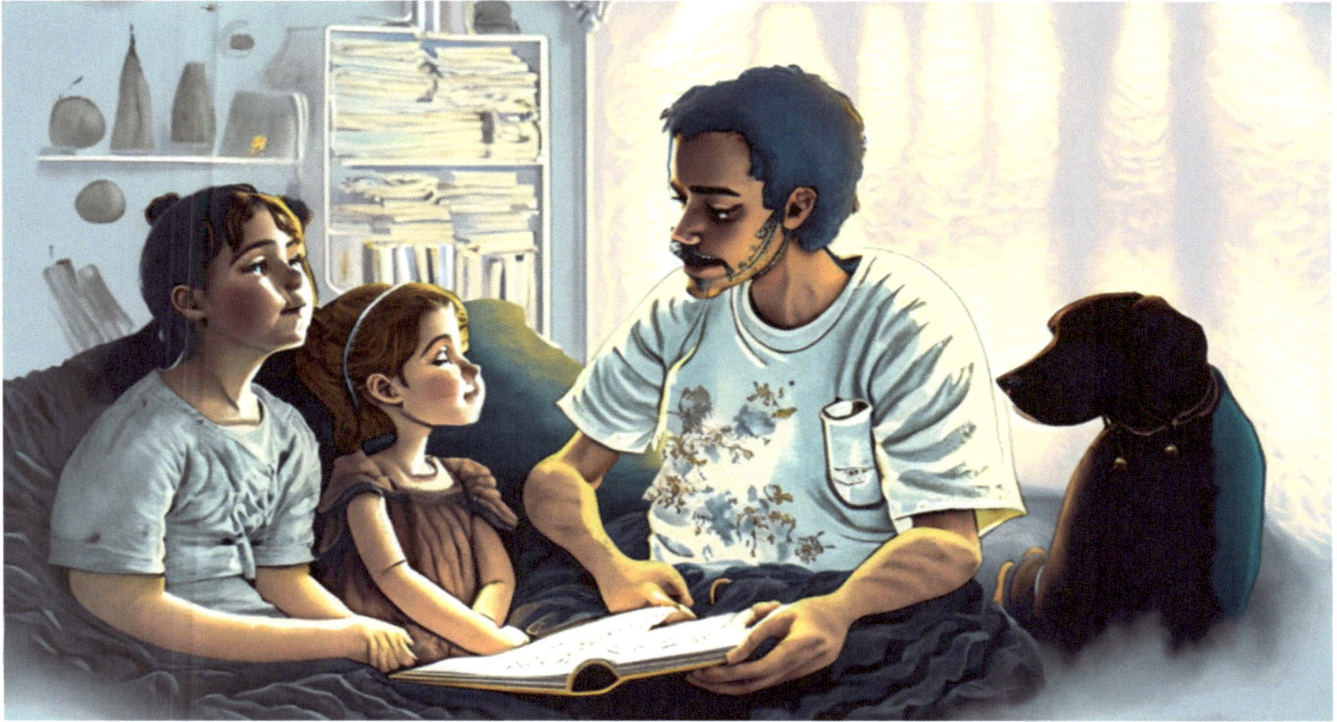

Canadian siblings, Saharsha, and Saumyaa, share a unique bond with their heritage, stronger than the roots of a maple tree! Though born far from their ancestral homeland, the stories and wisdom passed down through generations hold a special place in their hearts.

One day, Saharsha and Saumyaa come across their father deeply immersed in the Bhagavad Gita. Curiosity ignites in their eyes, and they approach him, eager to delve into the secrets of this ancient text and the profound wisdom it offers.

Saumyaa, with a thoughtful look, approached her dad. **"The Bhagavad-Gita,"** she began, *"it's been on my mind lately. Can you help me understand it better?"*

Her father's smile warmed the room. *"Of course, Saumyaa! It's a beautiful book, filled with wisdom that can guide anyone towards happiness and peace. It might be an ancient Hindu text, but its lessons are timeless."*

Dad chuckled, raising a finger playfully. *"Actually, the Bhagavad Gita isn't a massive book. It's just 18 chapters, with around 700 verses. That means you can learn a lot of valuable things without getting bogged down in endless reading. Even a few key teachings can make a big difference in your life!"*

Saumyaa's eyes sparkled with curiosity. "So, it's like a collection of wise sayings?"

Dad smiled. "Not exactly, Saumyaa. The title itself holds a deeper meaning. 'Bhagavad' means God or Supreme Being, and 'Gita' means song. So, the Bhagavad Gita translates to 'Song of God' or 'Sacred Song.' Some people believe that Lord Krishna himself sang these verses."

Saharsha piped in, tilting his head. "Lord Krishna? Like a superhero?"

Dad laughed. "Not quite, Saharsha. He's a central figure in the Hindu religion, often seen as a divine charioteer and guide. The Bhagavad Gita is actually set within a much larger story, an ancient Indian epic called the Mahabharata."

He closed his eyes for a moment, then began to paint a picture with his words "Imagine a time long ago, with two royal families locked in a bitter dispute. The Pandavas were known for their kindness and were the rightful heirs to the throne. But the Kauravas, led by the jealous Duryodhana, craved power and desired the kingdom for themselves."

"Peace talks failed," Dad continued, his voice dropping to a lower tone. "War loomed on the horizon, and the Pandavas faced a terrible choice: fight for their rightful land and their kin or choose peace even in the face of injustice. It was on this battlefield, amidst the chaos and uncertainty, that the story of the Bhagavad Gita unfolds."

"One of the Pandava brothers, Arjuna, a skilled warrior known for his bravery, found himself at a crossroads. He was filled with doubt and conflicted about fighting his own relatives. This is where Lord Krishna steps in, offering him not just military advice but also profound wisdom on duty, righteousness, and the path to enlightenment."

"He was forced to fight against his own loved ones - his teacher, friends, even family! The Bhagavad-Gita tells the story of his conversation with Lord Krishna, his charioteer and guide, who helps him overcome his inner struggle."

"The wisdom of the Gita teaches us the value of life and nonviolence, even in the darkest of times. It's a profound spiritual conversation that took place not in a temple, but right there on the battlefield."

Saharsha's eyes widened. *"Wow, Dad, that's incredible! Can you tell us more?"*

A grin spread across her father's face. "Absolutely, Saumyaa! How about a daily adventure? Each day, I can share one chapter of this story. Just make sure your schoolwork is done, and we'll begin tomorrow."

Saumyaa's smile rivaled the sun. "Thanks, Dad! I can't wait!"

# Chapter 1: Arjuna's Tough Choice

> ## *War Within: A Trailer for Chapter 1*

*Crimson dust swirls as Arjuna's chariot thunders across the battlefield! Arrows streak like flaming comets, warriors clash in a steel-blue storm. Can this legendary archer, clad in fiery orange, unleash his arrows on his own kin for a crown? Doubt, a serpent with eyes of fire, coils around his heart. But a golden light pierces the chaos, a voice whispers of honor and duty. Will Arjuna conquer his fear and unleash a storm of righteousness? Chapter 1: Witness the epic war within!*

Saharsha and Saumyaa huddled closer to their dad, their eyes wide with curiosity. "So, Dad," Saumyaa began, *"how did Lord Krishna and Arjuna end up talking on the battlefield?"*

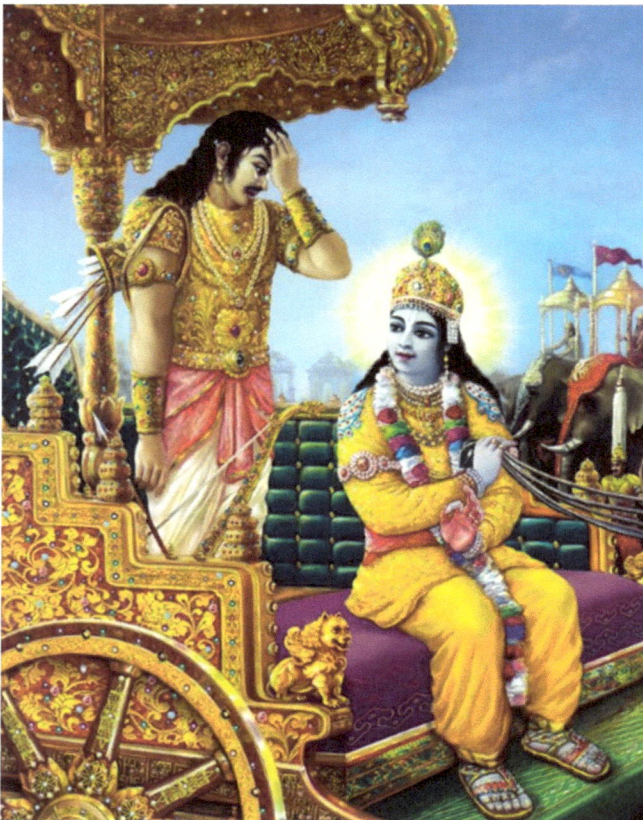

Their dad chuckled. "Ah, a great question! Imagine you have a big game coming up, maybe the championship match. You're feeling those butterflies in your tummy, right? Well, believe it or not, even super brave Prince Arjuna got them too, but not because he was scared of the fight!"

"He wasn't scared?" Saharsha asked, surprised.

"Not at all," Dad replied. "Arjuna was all set for a giant battle, ready to rumble alongside his best friend, Lord Krishna. They were like the coolest team ever! But when they got closer to the battlefield, something made Arjuna freeze in his tracks."

"What was it?" Saumyaa leaned in even closer.

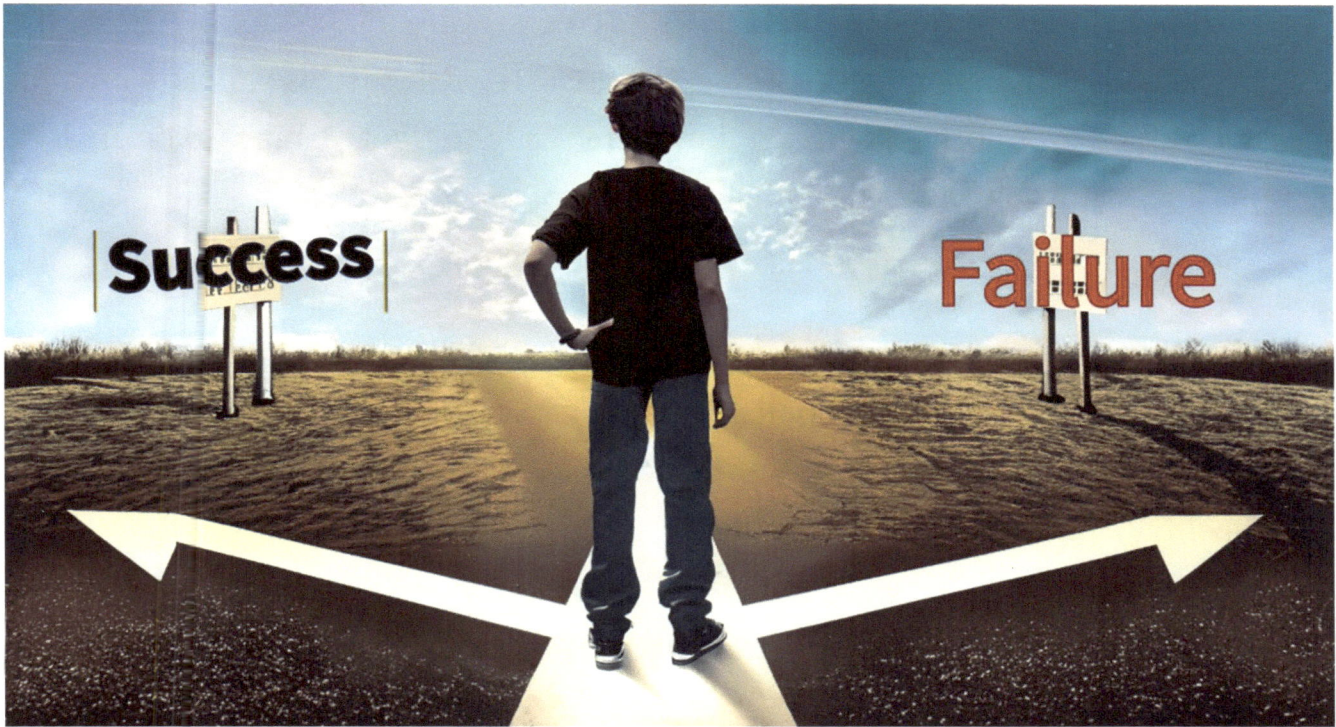

*A Hero's Journey Begins with a Choice*

"Taking a peek at the other side," Dad continued, "Arjuna saw something that made his heart sink. It was like a family reunion gone wrong! His grandpa, teachers, cousins, even some friends – all lined up against him!"

"Wait, he had to fight his own family?" Saharsha's eyes widened.

"Exactly," Dad said. "That's what made Arjuna feel so awful. How could he fight the people he loved? It just didn't feel right. This whole chapter is about Arjuna's struggle. Should he fight his loved ones or find another way to solve this big mess?"

"By the way," Dad added, "Arjuna's dad's older brother, Dhritarashtra, couldn't see because he was blind. So, he relied on his wise advisor, Sanjaya, to tell him everything that was happening on the battlefield, including this dramatic moment with Arjuna."

"So, what did Sanjaya tell Dhritarashtra?" Saumyaa pressed, eager to hear more.

Dad smiled. "Sanjaya described the scene. Duryodhana, Dhritarashtra s eldest son, was talking to their battle commander Dronacharya, who also happened to be the teacher of both Duryodhana and Arjuna. Then, the tension rose as warriors on both sides blew their war horns, signaling they were ready to fight. Sanjaya even spotted Krishna and Arjuna blowing their conches!"

"Cool!" Saharsha exclaimed.

"It was a big moment," Dad agreed. *"Arjuna's chariot, driven by Lord Krishna, carried a special flag. It depicted Lord Hanuman, the monkey god, a symbol of strength and devotion. He asked Krishna to stop right in the middle of the battlefield so he could get a closer look at the enemy – the Kauravas."*

"And then what?" Saumyaa prompted.

"Krishna stopped the chariot, and Arjuna took a good look," Dad said. "But what he saw filled him with dread. On both sides, he saw his own family – his grandpa, teachers, cousins, friends – all lined up ready to fight!"

"That's so sad," Saumyaa murmured.

"Exactly," Dad said. "Feeling heartbroken, Arjuna looked at Krishna and said, 'Krishna, all I see are my loved ones. Can we really fight and kill our own people for a kingdom? What good is a kingdom if it comes at the cost of killing my family and friends? This feels wrong, Krishna. I don't want to fight them.'"

Arjuna continued, filled with doubt, "Maybe the others are blinded by greed for power, but I won't be. I won't let greed and jealousy control me. I just can't fight them. It would be better if they attacked me, than for me to kill them."

"Sanjaya, witnessing Arjuna's despair, told Dhritarashtra, 'Your son, Arjuna, has dropped his bow and slumped in his chariot, filled with sadness.'"

## CHAPTER SUMMARY: ARJUNA'S TOUGH CHOICE

Arjuna, a brave prince, prepares for a huge fight with his wise friend Krishna by his side. But surprise! Instead of enemies, he sees his own family and friends on the opposing side!

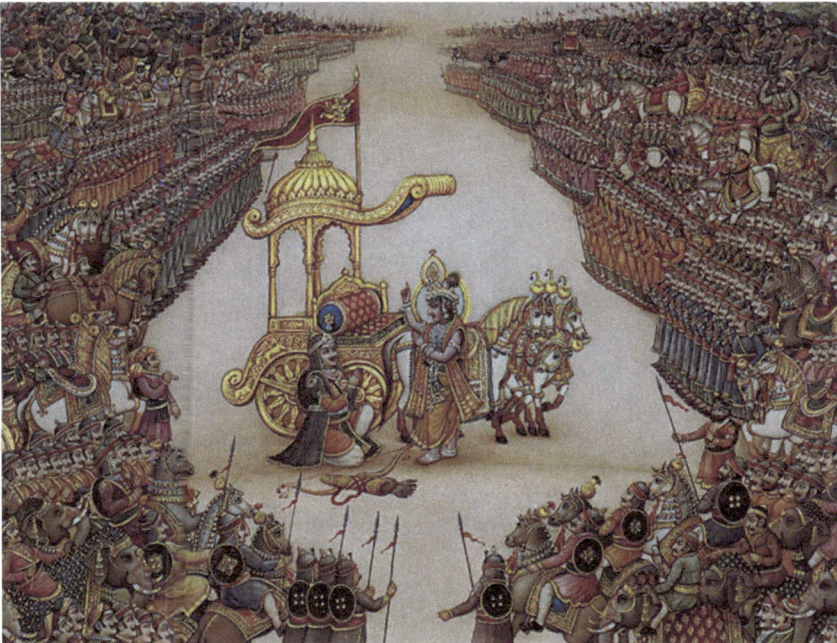

**Lord Krishna Emphasizing Action**

*"Arise, Arjuna! Shake off the shackles of fear and fight with righteousness as your guide. Victory lies not in the outcome, but in the righteous action."*

Arjuna is heartbroken. How can he fight the people he loves? Filled with doubt, he questions the whole war. Should he fight his family or find another solution?

We also meet Dhritarashtra, Arjuna's blind uncle, who relies on Sanjaya for battlefield updates. The war ignites due to a disagreement between the Pandavas (Arjuna's side) and the Kauravas (Dhritarashtra's sons). ⚔

This chapter sets the stage for an epic adventure! We meet the key players and witness Arjuna's difficult decision. Will he fight his loved ones? Stay tuned!

# Chapter 2: Krishna's Wise Advice

> ## The Chariot of Wisdom Rolls Forth – Lord Krishna's Wise Advice

**Arjuna, riddled with doubt**, stands amidst the carnage. Can righteous action coexist with fighting his own kin? *A celestial light descends! Krishna, the divine charioteer,* unveils the timeless wisdom of the Bhagavad Gita. *Prepare for a journey beyond the battlefield, where the secrets of karma, dharma, and the true Self are revealed.* Will Arjuna find clarity and purpose in Krishna's profound words? Chapter 2: Witness the Gita Revealed!

Dad smiled as he saw Saharsha and Saumyaa huddled together, their eyes wide with curiosity. "What's on your minds today, my little scholars?" he asked.

Saumyaa, ever the eager one, bounced in her seat. "Dad! Remember how Arjuna stopped his chariot and saw his family on the battlefield? Krishna explained all this deep stuff about the soul and stuff. Can you tell us about that?"

Dad chuckled. "Excellent question, Saumyaa! Chapter 2 of the Bhagavad Gita dives deeper into this concept. Here's what Krishna teaches Arjuna about the true Self, the Atman:"

## THE KNOWLEDGE OF THE ATMAN – KRISHNA'S WISE ADVICE

Dad pulled up a chair and sat beside them. "Imagine you have a favorite doll; one you've played with for years. But then, you get a brand new, super cool one. You might still love your old doll, but you're excited to play with the new one, right?"

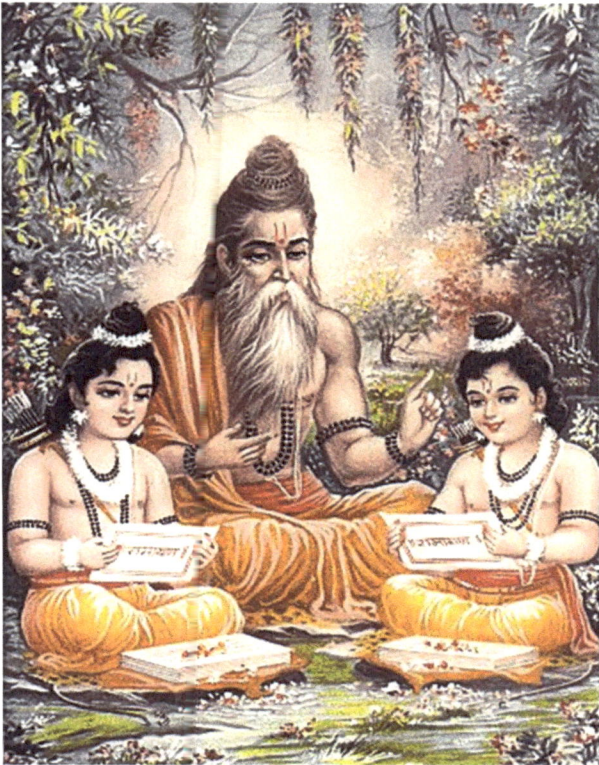

Saharsha's brow furrowed. "But what does that have to do with Arjuna?"

"Think of the body as the doll," Dad explained. "Our bodies change and grow old, just like a doll gets worn and tattered. But inside, there's something else, something that never gets old. That's the Atman, like the you that stays the same even as your doll changes."

"So, we're not just our bodies?" Saumyaa gasped.

"Exactly!" Dad said. "The Atman is the real us, the eternal part that goes on a journey from one body to another, just like you might move from your old dollhouse to a new, bigger one."

Saumyaa's eyes sparkled. "So, when people die, their Atman just goes and finds a new body?"

Dad nodded. "That's the idea! It's like changing clothes. You take off your old outfit and put on a new one. The Atman is like the you that stays the same underneath all those clothes."

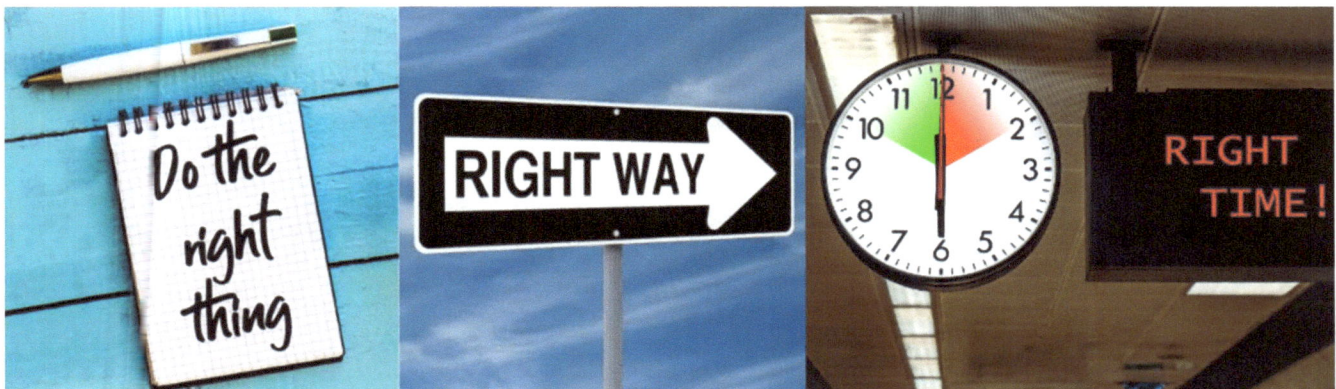

## ARJUNA'S CONFLICT

Saharsha chimed in, "But why was Arjuna so worried about fighting his relatives then?"

"That's a great question," Dad said. "Arjuna cared about his family very much. He saw them on the other side of the battlefield, and it made him sad to think he might have to hurt them. But Krishna reminded him that the Atman, the real person inside, can't be hurt."

"It's like if your dollhouse got broken," Dad continued. "You might feel sad, but you know you can still play with your dolls in another house, right?"

Saumyaa seemed to ponder this. "So, even though Arjuna's grandfather's body might get hurt, his Atman would be, okay?"

"Exactly!" Dad said. "Krishna was teaching Arjuna that it's important to focus on our duty and what's right, even if it's difficult. Arjuna's duty was to fight for what was right, and Krishna was helping him see that fighting wouldn't harm the Atman, the true self, of anyone involved."

"Wow," Saharsha said, a thoughtful look on his face. "That's hard to think about."

Dad ruffled Saharsha's hair. "It is, isn't it? But it's an important idea. Chapter 2 of the Bhagavad Gita lays the foundation for understanding the core concepts of Karma Yoga (yoga of action) and the message of the entire book."

## CHAPTER SUMMARY: KRISHNA'S WISE ADVICE ABOUT YOU

### The Real You (Atma)

This chapter dives into who we truly are, deeper than our bodies. Imagine your favorite well-loved toy. Now picture a brand new one! You might still cherish the old one, but the new one sparks excitement.

Krishna uses this analogy to explain the Atman. Our bodies, like the old toy, change and grow. But within, there's a special, unchanging part - the Atman. It's the essence of you that remains constant throughout life's changes.

So, the Atman is the real us? Yes! The Atman is like you moving from a dollhouse to a bigger one. When our bodies grow old, the Atman simply moves on to a new "body," just like putting on new clothes!

This explains Arjuna's worry. He didn't want to fight his family. But Krishna reminds him that the Atman, the true self, can't be harmed. It's like a broken dollhouse; you can still play with the dolls in a new one.

While fighting was difficult, Krishna emphasized doing the right thing, even if it's hard. Arjuna's duty was to fight for what was right. Krishna explains that fighting wouldn't harm the Atman, the true self, of anyone involved.

This chapter is the foundation for a grand adventure! It helps us understand who we truly are and that a special part of us remains constant throughout life's journey. Pretty cool, right?

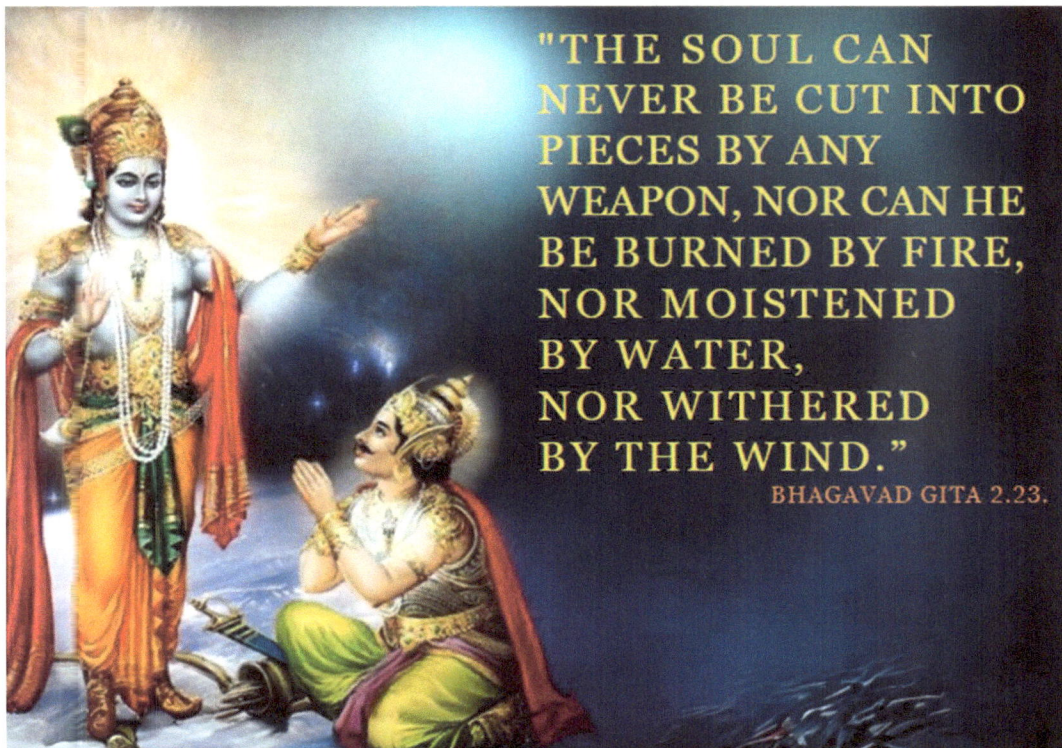

"THE SOUL CAN NEVER BE CUT INTO PIECES BY ANY WEAPON, NOR CAN HE BE BURNED BY FIRE, NOR MOISTENED BY WATER, NOR WITHERED BY THE WIND."
BHAGAVAD GITA 2.23.

# Chapter 3: Karma Yoga - Doing Your Best

"

## *Karma Yoga – Unleash Your Inner Hero!*

*Mysterious whispers fill the air as Saumyaa and Saharsha huddle closer to Dad. A glowing book unfolds, revealing a fantastical tale: The Magic Mango Tree! Its shimmering fruit grants wishes, but only to those with pure hearts. Enter Ravi, a boy consumed by selfish desires. Will he pluck the fruit for personal gain? Suddenly, a wise woman appears! She introduces Mohan, a kind farmer seeking rain to save his village. A choice unfolds, shimmering with golden light. Can Ravi overcome his ego? Chapter 3: Witness Karma Yoga in action! Unleash the hero within and discover the magic of helping others!*

After finishing their homework, chores, and a delicious dinner, Saumyaa and Saharsha snuggled up next to their dad, their eyes sparkling with curiosity. "Dad, can you tell us more about the Bhagavad Gita?" they asked eagerly.

Dad smiled warmly and nodded. "Today, we'll explore Chapter 3, which dives into **Karma Yoga, the 'path of action.'** It's a beautiful way to find happiness by using your talents to help others."

## WHAT IS KARMA YOGA?

"Karma Yoga is all about doing your duties and actions with a selfless attitude," Dad explained. "It means performing your work, big or small, as a service to others, without being attached to the results or expecting anything in return."

Saumyaa tilted her head. "But don't we usually do things to get rewarded or praised?"

"That's a common way of thinking," Dad replied. "But Karma Yoga teaches us to shift our mindset. Instead of acting for personal gain, we act out of love and concern for the well-being of others."

## WHY DO GOOD DEEDS MATTER?

Saumyaa, ever the inquisitive one, bounced in her seat. "But Dad, why can't we just do things we enjoy? Why does Krishna say we have to control our desires?"

Dad chuckled and ruffled her curls. "Ah, that's a wise question, my dear. Imagine you have a box filled with your favorite chocolates. If you gobbled them all up at once, you'd likely feel sick! When we act only on our desires, without thinking of others, it can lead to problems. But Karma Yoga teaches us a different way."

## TWO PATHS TO HAPPINESS

"You know how there's more than one trail to reach the top of a mountain?" Dad continued. "Similarly, the Gita teaches different paths to happiness. Chapter 2 explored Jnana Yoga, the path of knowledge. Today, we'll learn about Karma Yoga, which is perfect for most people."

## FINDING YOUR CALLING THROUGH HELPING OTHERS

Saharsha chimed in, his eyes wide with curiosity. "So, is Karma Yoga about helping others? Like how Uncle Rohan volunteers at the animal shelter on weekends?"

"Precisely!" Dad exclaimed. "Uncle Rohan does his duty without expecting anything in return. That's Karma Yoga in action! You see, every job, big or small, can be a way to serve others. Karma Yoga is about using your skills and talents to make the world a better place, whether you become a doctor, a teacher, an artist, or anything else."

"Even something as simple as doing your chores at home with a positive attitude is an act of Karma Yoga," Dad added. "Because you're helping to make your family's life a little easier, without expecting praise or rewards."

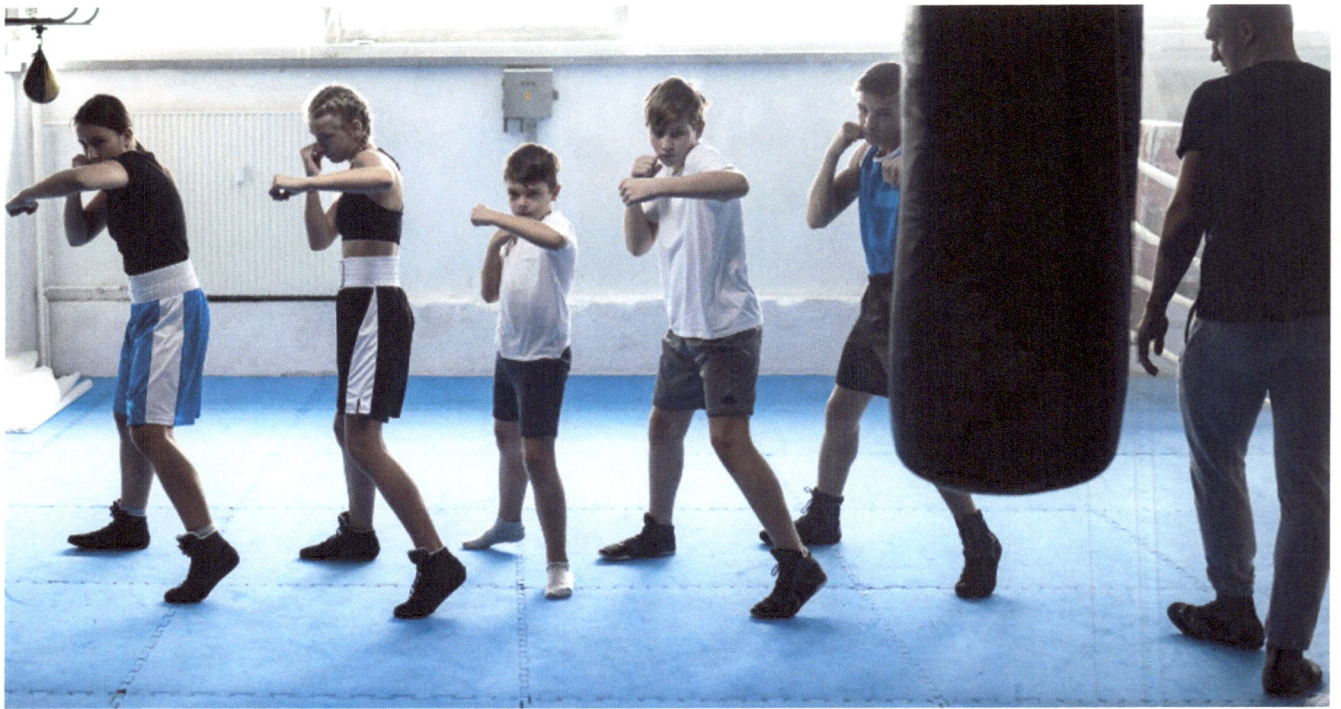

*Practice with Dedication & Focus*

## THE TALE OF THE MAGIC MANGO TREE

"There's an enchanting story that helps explain Karma Yoga," Dad said, his voice taking on a storyteller's cadence. "In a faraway land, nestled between snow-capped mountains, stood a magical mango tree. Its fruit was said to grant your greatest desire, but only if your heart was pure."

Saumyaa gasped, her eyes widening like saucers. "Wow! What kind of desires could it grant?"

Dad leaned closer, his voice hushed with wonder. "All sorts of desires, my dear. Some people wished for riches beyond imagination, while others yearned for fame and power. But the key was how you used the fruit's magic."

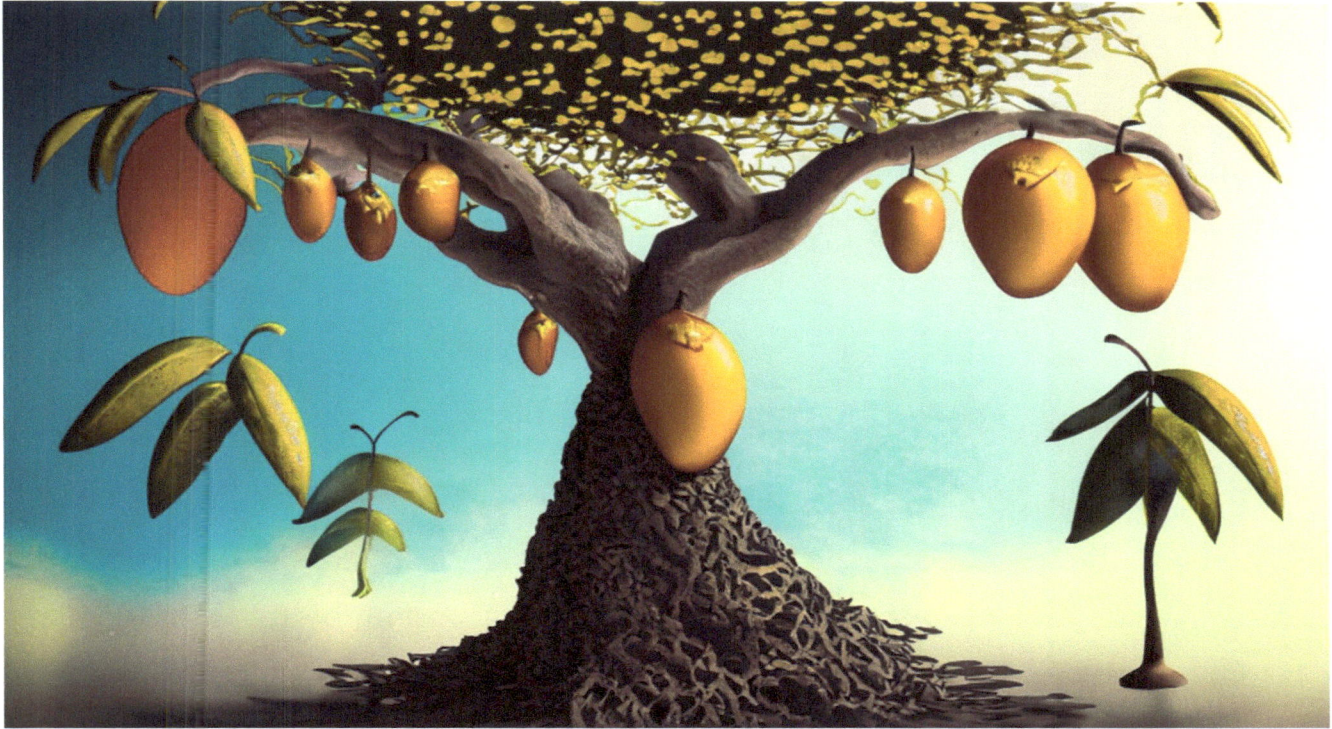

## SELFISH DESIRES VS. SELFLESS SERVICE

"Once upon a time, there was a young man named Ravi. He dreamed of a life filled with fancy things and being the center of attention, so he embarked on a long journey to find the magical mango tree."

"Did he find it?" Saharsha asked, his breath caught in his throat.

"He did," Dad nodded solemnly. "After many adventures, Ravi found the tree and reached for the last magical mango, hoping it would make him rich and famous forever."

"But just as he was about to pluck the fruit, a wise old woman appeared and stopped him. 'Young traveler,' she said, 'are you sure that getting everything you desire will truly make you happy forever?'"

"What did Ravi say?" Saumyaa asked, her eyes wide with anticipation.

"Ravi hesitated, suddenly unsure of himself," Dad said. "Then, the wise woman introduced him to another traveler, a kind farmer named Mohan."

## TRUE HAPPINESS COMES FROM HELPING OTHERS

"Mohan wasn't interested in riches or fame," Dad explained, his voice soft and reverent. "His village was suffering from a terrible drought, and their crops were dying. Mohan hoped the magic mango could bring rain to save his people from starving."

"Oh no!" Saumyaa gasped. "That's so much more important than getting toys and jewels!"

Dad nodded sagely. "Indeed, my dear. Seeing Mohan's kindness and selflessness, Ravi realized his own wishes were selfish. Without hesitation, he stepped aside and let Mohan take the magic mango."

"And do you know what happened next?" Dad asked, his eyes twinkling. "The magic mango, when shared by Mohan, brought life-giving rain to his village, saving countless lives."

## TRUE HAPPINESS THROUGH KARMA YOGA

"So, helping others is the real key to happiness?" Saharsha asked thoughtfully.

"Precisely!" Dad said, beaming with pride. "That's the heart of Karma Yoga. It's about doing your very best and using your talents to serve others, without expecting anything in return. Just like Mohan, when you focus on helping those in need, you'll find true happiness and fulfillment."

## THE POWER OF YOUR THOUGHTS

Dad concluded, "Remember, my dear ones, your mind is a powerful force. Before you act on a desire, think about how it might affect others. Choose kindness and service, and you'll be well on your way to becoming true Karma Yogis, just like the wise sages of the Gita."

Saumyaa and Saharsha gazed at their dad with newfound wonder, their hearts filled with the timeless wisdom of the Bhagavad Gita, and a desire to use their talents to make the world a better place.

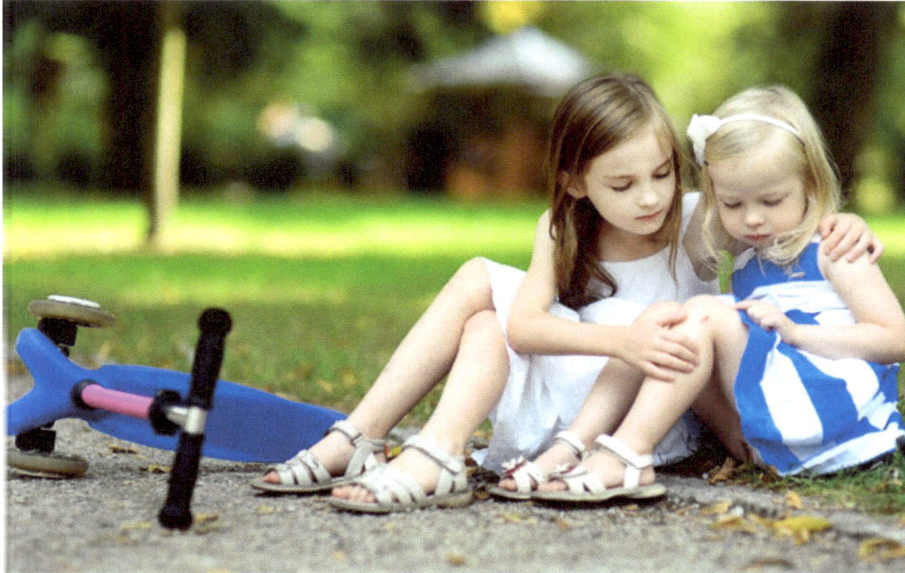

## SAUMYAA AND SAHARSHA'S EVERYDAY KARMA YOGA QUESTIONS:

1. **Saumyaa:** *Dad, in school, we sometimes have to work on group projects. How can I use Karma Yoga when some people don't do their part?*

**Dad:** That's a great question, Saumyaa! Karma Yoga teaches us to do our best, no matter what others do. You can try to communicate calmly with your group members and offer to help them understand the project. But ultimately, you can only control your own actions. Do your assigned part to the best of your ability and remember, a cheerful outlook can be contagious!

2. **Saharsha:** *Sometimes I get frustrated with my homework. Can doing homework be Karma Yoga?*

**Dad:** Absolutely, Saharsha! Learning is a valuable skill that helps you grow and understand the world around you. When you put effort into your homework, you're not just doing it for a grade, you're investing in your own future. That's a perfect example of Karma Yoga – doing your duty with dedication.

3. **Saumyaa:** *At home, we sometimes have chores. Can doing chores be Karma Yoga too?*

**Dad:** Definitely, Saumyaa! Chores help keep your home clean and organized, making it a more comfortable place for everyone. When you do your chores without complaining, you're contributing to the well-being of your family. That's a great way to practice Karma Yoga!

4. **Saharsha:** *Dad, sometimes I feel shy to help others, even though I want to. How can I overcome that shyness and practice Karma Yoga?*

**Dad:** It's okay to feel shy sometimes, Saharsha. But even small acts of kindness can make a big difference. Maybe you can start by offering to help someone who looks like they might need it. Or you could smile at someone who seems sad. Even a small gesture can brighten someone's day and that's a way of practicing Karma Yoga.

5. **Saumyaa & Saharsha (together):** *Dad, can we use Karma Yoga to make new friends?*

**Dad:** You might be surprised, but yes! Karma Yoga is about building positive relationships. By being kind, helpful, and respectful to others, you're creating a foundation for friendship. People are naturally drawn to those who are positive and supportive. So, keep practicing Karma Yoga, and you'll find yourself attracting good friends who share your values.

6. **Saumyaa:** *Dad, the story showed Mohan getting the magic mango because his wish was selfless. But what if someone has a strong desire to help others, but they don't know how to yet? Can that still be Karma Yoga?*

**Dad:** That's a wonderful question, Saumyaa! Absolutely. Karma Yoga isn't just about the outcome, it's also about the intention behind your actions. Even if you're still learning how to help others, the genuine desire to do good is a part of Karma Yoga. As you learn and grow, you'll find ways to use your skills and talents to make a positive impact.

7. **Saharsha:** *Sometimes it's hard to be helpful, especially when someone is being mean. Can Karma Yoga still work then?*

**Dad:** That's a tricky one, Saharsha. Karma Yoga is about acting with kindness and service, even when it's challenging. Maybe helping someone who's mean means showing them patience or understanding. It might not always be easy, but by staying calm and respectful, you might inspire them to act differently.

8. **Saumyaa & Saharsha (together):** *But what if helping others takes a lot of time and effort? Won't we get tired of doing things for other people all the time?*

**Dad:** That's a good point! It's important to find a balance between helping others and taking care of yourself. Karma Yoga doesn't mean neglecting your own needs. Listen to your body and mind. Take breaks when you need them, and remember, even small acts of kindness can make a big difference.

9. **Saharsha:** *The story said the magic mango helped the whole village. Can we really make a big difference by ourselves?*

**Dad:** You might be surprised, Saharsha! Even small acts of kindness can have a ripple effect. Helping a friend, cleaning up your neighborhood, or simply being kind to someone who's having a bad day – it all adds up. When many people act with compassion, the positive impact can be enormous.

10. **Saumyaa:** *Dad, is Karma Yoga just about helping people? Can it be about taking care of the environment too?*

**Dad:** Absolutely, Saumyaa! The world around us is full of life that needs our care. Recycling, planting trees, or even just being mindful not to waste resources are all ways to practice Karma Yoga. Taking care of the planet is a way of serving something bigger than ourselves.

11. **Saumyaa:** *Dad, why can't we just do things we enjoy? Why does Krishna say we have to control our desires?*

**Dad:** That's a great question, Saumyaa! Imagine you have a delicious box of chocolates. You might gobble them all up right away, but then you'd feel sick! When we only act on our desires, it can lead to problems. Karma Yoga teaches us to find a balance and use our skills to help others, which brings a different kind of happiness.

12. **Saharsha:** *So, is Karma Yoga like helping others? Like how Uncle Rohan volunteers at the anima shelter on weekends?*

**Dad:** Exactly, Saharsha! Uncle Rohan does his duty without expecting anything in return. That's Karma Yoga in action! Every job, big or small, can be a way to serve others. Maybe you'll be a doctor, a teacher, or an artist – you can use your skills to help people in your own way.

13.  **Saumyaa:** *But wouldn't people work harder if they wanted a reward?*

**Dad:** Maybe in the short term. But true happiness comes from doing good for others, not just getting things for yourself. A Karma Yogi does their best work because they know it helps the world around them. It's like planting a seed – you take care of it, and it grows into something beautiful that benefits everyone.

14.  **Saharsha:** *So, how can we know what our duty is?*

**Dad:** That's a great question too! Sometimes, your duty might be your schoolwork, helping around the house, or being kind to your friends. As you get older, you'll discover your talents and passions. Use those to help others – that's your Karma Yoga!

15.  **Saumyaa:** *The story had a magic mango tree. Are there magic things that help us do Karma Yoga?*

**Dad:** Not exactly, Saumyaa. The magic in the story represents the power of helping others. When you do good deeds, it creates a ripple effect of happiness, just like the rain brought life to the village. You don't need magic; your kindness and hard work are all you need to make a difference!

16.  **Saumyaa:** *Dad, the story showed that Mohan's selfless wish brought him happiness. But what if someone sacrifices their own happiness to help others? Is that still Karma Yoga?*

**Dad:** That's a profound question, Saumyaa. True happiness comes from living a life of purpose and service. While there will be times when helping others requires sacrifice, the fulfillment you get from making a positive difference can be much deeper than personal happiness. Karma Yoga encourages us to find a balance between our own needs and the needs of others.

17.  **Saumyaa:** *Dad, the story was about getting a magic fruit. But in real life, what if our actions don't always have positive outcomes? Can Karma Yoga still work?*

**Dad:** That's a great point, Saumyaa. Karma Yoga focuses on the act of service, not necessarily the outcome. Even if things don't go as planned, the intention behind your actions matters. You can't control everything, but you can control your own choices. By acting with kindness and compassion, you contribute to a better world, even if the results aren't always immediate or obvious.

**Dad** smiled warmly. "Those are some fantastic questions, Saumyaa and Saharsha! You've really grasped the essence of Karma Yoga. Remember, even small acts of kindness can make a big difference. Keep practicing, and you'll find happiness and fulfillment in serving others."

He glanced at the clock. "Wow, it's getting late! Tomorrow's a school day, and we have another exciting chapter of the Bhagavad Gita to explore. How about we get some rest and pick up our story then?"

**Saharsha** yawned dramatically. *"Sounds good, Dad. Thanks for the story!"*

**Saumyaa** stretched. *"Goodnight, Dad. And goodnight, Karma Yoga!"*

**Dad** chuckled. *"Goodnight, you two. Sweet dreams filled with helping others and making the world a better place!"*

## CHAPTER SUMMARY: KARMA YOGA – DOING YOUR BEST

Chapter 3 explores Karma Yoga, also known as the "path of action." Here are the key takeaways:

- **Don't be ruled by desires:** Just like overindulging in sweets, acting only on desires can lead to problems. Karma Yoga teaches us to control our desires for true happiness.

- **Two paths to happiness:** There's no single path! Similar to climbing a mountain, there are different ways to find happiness. Karma Yoga is a practical approach, perfect for most people.

- **Helping others is the key:** Karma Yoga is all about serving others. Whether it's volunteering like Uncle Rohan or using your talents like becoming a doctor, helping others brings true joy.

- **Doing your best matters more than rewards:** While rewards can motivate us sometimes, true happiness comes from doing good for others. A Karma Yogi focuses on putting their best effort into everything they do, knowing it contributes to a better world.

- **Control your thoughts, choose kindness:** Our thoughts are powerful! Before acting on a desire, consider how it might affect others. Choose kindness and service over selfishness to become a true Karma Yogi.

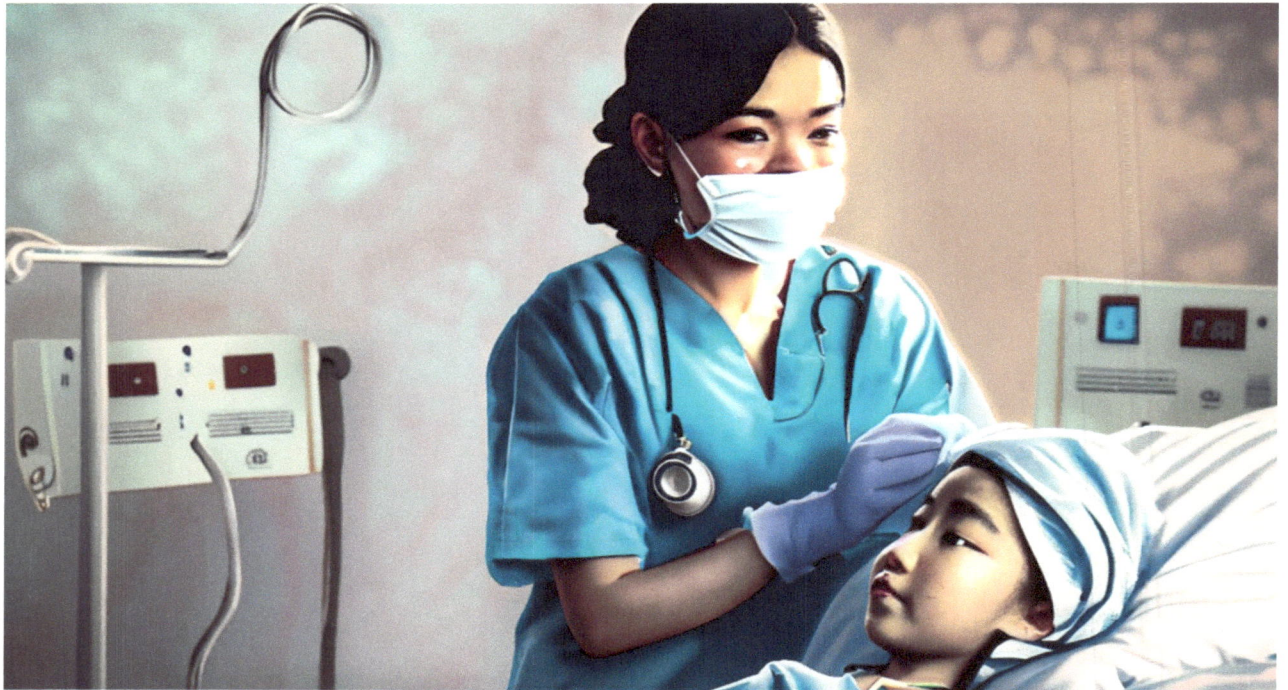

# Chapter 4: The Soul Inside Us

"

## *The Shimmering Soul – A Journey Within*

*Ever wondered what lies beyond the physical? Saumyaa and Saharsha embark on a magical quest in Chapter 4! Join them as the Bhagavad Gita unveils the secrets of the Shimmering Soul, the essence within. Is it a tiny light, or something grander? Explore the cycle of karma and the power of selfless acts. Can you break free and reach enlightenment? Chapter 4: Witness the journey inward and discover the hero within yourself!*

Dad: Have you two finished your homework for tonight? Saharsha: (Sighs) Almost, Dad. Just a few more math problems to go. Saumyaa: I'm all done with mine! Can we start reading the Bhagavad Gita now? I'm so excited!

Dad chuckled, his eyes twinkling with warmth. "Of course, Saumyaa! Tonight's chapter is titled **'The Soul Inside Us,'** and it's a question that has captivated the hearts and minds of people for thousands of years, even before this ancient book was written."

Saharsha perked up, intrigued. "Cool! So, what's the answer? Do we all have tiny souls inside us like glowing marbles?"

Dad smiled and ruffled Saharsha's hair affectionately. "Not quite, my curious one. The soul isn't something physical we can hold in our hands. It's the essence of who we truly are, the spark that makes us alive and connects us to the divine."

Saumyaa's eyes widened with wonder. "So, it's like the energy in our batteries that keeps us going, but more magical?"

"That's an insightful analogy, Saumyaa!" Dad exclaimed. "But the soul is more than just energy. It's what gives us our unique personalities, emotions, and consciousness – the qualities that make us human, different from even the most advanced robots."

Saharsha furrowed his brow, deep in thought. "So, what happens to our soul when our battery, I mean, our body, runs out?"

Dad's expression grew solemn as he nodded. "That's a profound question, Saharsha, one that philosophers and spiritual seekers have been grappling with for centuries. The Bhagavad Gita teaches us about the Atman, the true Self. It says the Atman is eternal, like a flame that can never be extinguished."

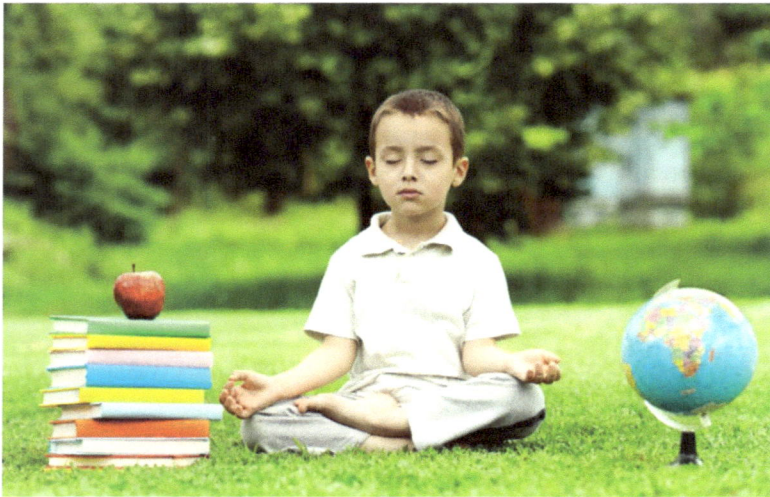

*Lord Krishna describes the atman as the true self, the permanent and unchanging essence that resides within each living being.*

*Bhagavad Gita, Chapter 2.12*

Saumyaa gasped, her eyes sparkling with curiosity. "So, our soul just keeps going on and on, even after we die?"

"That's the idea, Saumyaa," Dad replied gently. "But where it goes and what happens next depends on what you believe. Different religions and philosophies have different perspectives on the journey of the soul."

Saharsha leaned forward, utterly engrossed. "Do they all talk about the soul too?"

Dad nodded. "Indeed, Saharsha. In Christianity, for instance, they believe the soul is a gift from God, separate from the physical body. In Buddhism, there's a concept of rebirth and reincarnation, but not a permanent, unchanging soul. It's a complex and fascinating topic."

Saumyaa's brow furrowed as she pondered this. "Wow, so many different ideas! How do we know which one is right?"

Dad smiled warmly, his eyes filled with wisdom. "There's no easy answer, my dear Saumyaa. Perhaps the most important thing is to believe in something that resonates with your heart and gives your life a sense of meaning and purpose."

Saharsha nodded slowly, his expression thoughtful. "And maybe understand ourselves better, too?"

"Precisely, Saharsha!" Dad exclaimed. "This search for self-knowledge is at the heart of many spiritual practices. By understanding our own souls, we can live a life of deeper fulfillment and inner peace."

Saumyaa's eyes lit up with realization. "That's why people meditate, isn't it? To connect with their souls?"

Dad beamed, pride shining in his eyes. "You're absolutely right, Saumyaa! Meditation and other spiritual practices can help us quiet our minds and connect with that deeper essence within ourselves – our Atman, our true Self."

Saharsha let out a long exhale. "Whew, this is a lot to think about, Dad!"

Dad chuckled warmly. "Take your time, my son. There are no right or wrong answers here. The important thing is to keep asking questions and exploring these profound ideas with an open heart and mind."

Saumyaa's eyes shone with enthusiasm. "Can we learn more about different beliefs about the soul next time? And maybe some stories to help us understand better?"

"Of course, Saumyaa!" Dad exclaimed. "There's a whole world of fascinating tales and wisdom waiting to be discovered.

# THE TALE OF THE WISE OLD SAGE

Saumyaa's eyes lit up with enthusiasm. "Dad, you mentioned there were fascinating tales about the soul from different beliefs. Can you share one with us?"

Dad smiled warmly. "Of course, my dear. Let me tell you the Tale of the Wise Old Sage."

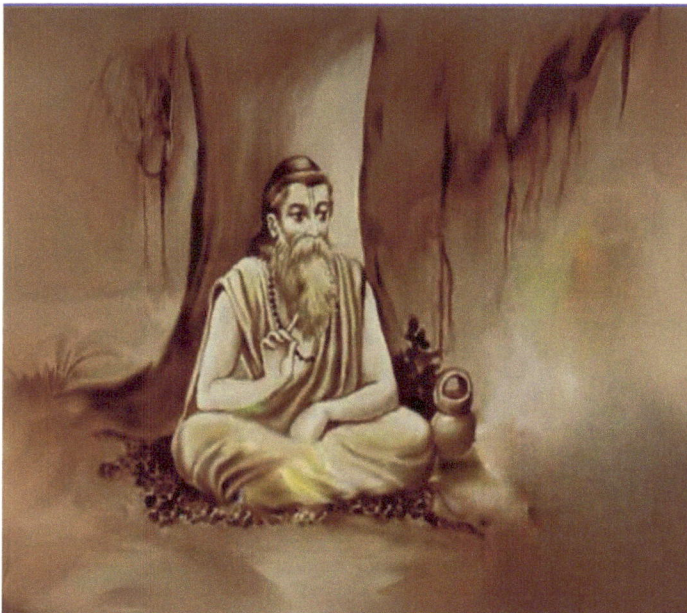

Saharsha leaned forward, his eyes wide with curiosity. "Ooh, this sounds exciting!"

Dad began, his voice taking on a storyteller's cadence. "In a peaceful village nestled amidst lush green hills and surrounded by fragrant jasmine fields, there lived a wise old sage named Guruji..."

Saumyaa interrupted, "What was Guruji like, Dad?"

"Ah, Guruji was a remarkable soul," Dad replied. "His kind eyes sparkled with ancient wisdom, and his gentle smile radiated a warmth that could melt even the coldest of hearts. He was revered by all the villagers, who sought his guidance on matters of the soul and spirituality."

Saharsha nodded, hanging on to every word. "I can picture him already. So, what happened next?"

Dad continued, "One crisp morning, as the village awoke to the melodious chirping of birds, the villagers gathered around Guruji's humble abode, a simple dwelling adorned with vibrant marigold garlands. Among them was a young boy named Anand, his eyes wide with curiosity."

"Guruji emerged, his white robes rustling softly in the cool breeze, and greeted the villagers with a benevolent nod. Anand stepped forward, his small voice wavering with nervousness. 'Guruji,' he asked, 'what is the soul, and where does it reside?'"

Saumyaa gasped, "That's such an important question! What did Guruji say?"

"Guruji's weathered face broke into a warm smile, and he motioned for Anand to sit closer. The other villagers leaned in, eager to hear the sage's wisdom. Guruji began to narrate a tale that had been passed down through generations, his voice rich and captivating."

## THE ENLIGHTENMENT OF PRINCE SIDDHARTHA

Dad paused, creating a moment of suspense, before resuming, "Many years ago, in a distant kingdom, there reigned a noble king…"

**King Suddhodana**, ruler of the **Shakya clan**, enjoyed prosperity and power. His palace gleamed with gold, and the fragrant gardens bloomed year-round. Yet, hidden behind the opulence, a deeper longing stirred within him—a desire to understand the essence of existence.

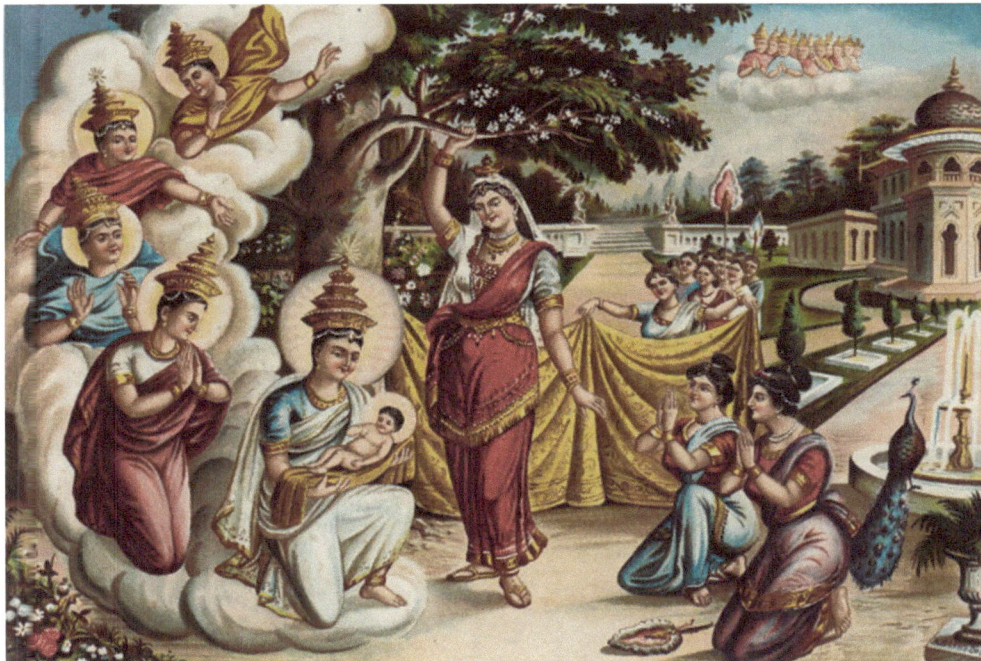

One moonlit night, as the stars whispered their secrets, Queen **Maya** dreamt of a white elephant—an auspicious sign. Soon after, she discovered she was with child. The kingdom rejoiced, for this child was destined to be extraordinary.

And so, on a spring morning, in the sacred groves of **Lumbini**, Queen Maya gave birth to a son. The earth seemed to hold its breath as the infant emerged. His skin glowed like polished sandalwood, and his eyes held ancient wisdom. The gods themselves rejoiced, for this child was no ordinary prince.

They named him **Siddhartha**, which means "he who achieves his goals." The prophecy whispered that he would either become a great king or a world-renowned sage.

As Siddhartha grew, he reveled in princely pleasures—the silk robes, the jeweled ornaments, and the sweet melodies that echoed through the palace. But even amidst this splendor, a restlessness gnawed at his heart. He wondered about the world beyond the palace walls—the suffering, impermanence, and the elusive truth that lay hidden.

One day, Siddhartha ventured beyond the palace gates. There, he encountered an old man, bent with age, leaning on a staff. His wrinkled face told stories of joy and sorrow, love and loss. Siddhartha's heart trembled. He had never seen such vulnerability.

Next, he met a sick man, writhing in pain. Disease had ravaged his body, leaving him frail and feeble. Siddhartha's youthful vigor suddenly felt fragile.

Lastly, he encountered a funeral procession. A lifeless body lay on a bier, surrounded by mourners. The air smelled of incense and grief. Siddhartha pondered the impermanence of existence—the fleeting nature of life itself.

These encounters shook him to the core. The palace walls could no longer contain his curiosity. Siddhartha yearned for answers—to unravel the mysteries of birth, aging, sickness, and death. His heart whispered of a deeper purpose, beyond princely duties.

And so, like a lotus seeking sunlight, Prince Siddhartha embarked on a quest—a journey that would lead him to enlightenment, compassion, and the path of awakening. He wandered through forests and mountains, seeking answers to the mysteries of existence.

After years of rigorous meditation and contemplation, Prince Siddhartha attained enlightenment under the Bodhi tree. He realized that the soul, or Atman, resides within each living being, transcending the physical body and connecting all living creatures to the divine cosmic energy.

As Guruji concluded the tale, he looked at Anand and the other villagers with warmth in his eyes. "Just like Prince Siddhartha, each one of us carries the divine spark of the soul within us," Guruji explained. "It is the essence of our being, guiding us on our journey of self-discovery and spiritual awakening."

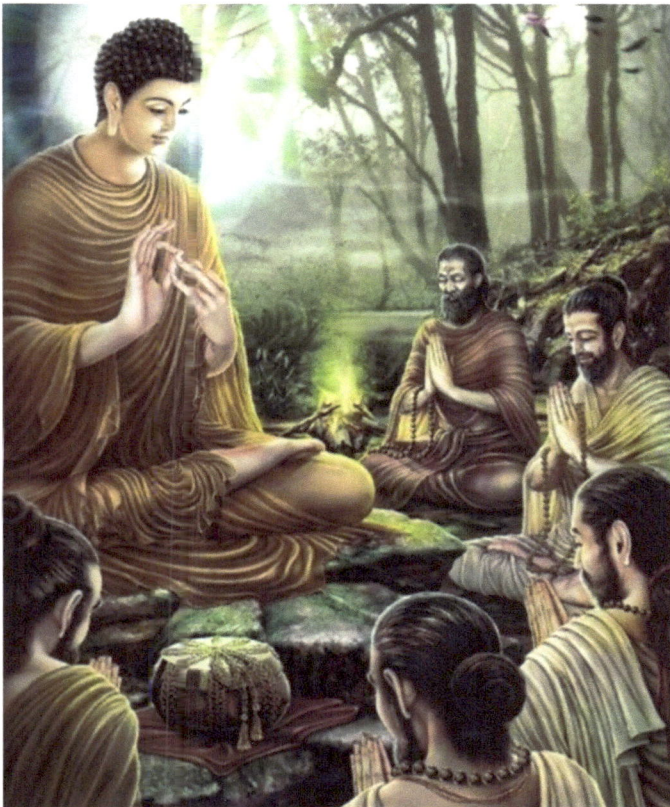

*(Gautam Buddha with his disciples)*

The villagers listened intently to Guruji's words, feeling a sense of awe and reverence for the profound wisdom hidden within the depths of their own souls. And from that day forward, they embarked on a journey of inner exploration, seeking to connect with the eternal soul that resided within each of them.

After narrating the profound tale, Dad looked at Saumyaa and Saharsha with a twinkle in his eye. "As Guruji concluded the story, he gazed upon the enraptured faces of the villagers, their eyes shining with wonder and reverence..."

Saharsha was spellbound. "Wow, what an incredible story! I can just imagine the villagers' reactions."

Dad nodded sagely. "Indeed, my son. 'Just like Prince Siddhartha, each one of us carries the divine spark of the soul within us,' Guruji explained, his voice resonating with conviction. 'It is the essence of our being, guiding us on our journey of self-discovery and spiritual awakening.'"

Saumyaa's eyes shone with newfound understanding. "So, the story taught them about the eternal nature of the soul, and how it connects us all to the divine."

"Precisely, Saumyaa," Dad said, beaming with pride. "The villagers sat in silence, their hearts filled with a newfound appreciation for the profound wisdom hidden within the depths of their own souls. And from that day forward, they embarked on a journey of inner exploration, seeking to connect with the eternal Atman that resided within each of them."

## THE STORY OF EKALAVYA

"There once lived a young boy named Ekalavya, born into a humble family of forest dwellers," Dad began, his voice taking on a storyteller's cadence. "Though his circumstances were modest, Ekalavya harbored a dream that burned brighter than a thousand suns – to become the greatest archer the land had ever seen."

Saharsha's eyes widened with excitement. "Wow, that's an ambitious dream for someone from such a simple background!"

Dad nodded sagely. "Indeed, my son. But Ekalavya's determination knew no bounds. You see, in those days, the revered archery teacher, Dronacharya, only accepted princes and nobility as his students, turning away all others."

Saumyaa frowned, her brow furrowing with indignation. "That's not fair! Ekalavya shouldn't be left out just because he's not royalty."

"You're absolutely right, Saumyaa," Dad agreed. "But Ekalavya refused to let societal norms and traditions hold him back. With unwavering focus and ingenuity, he crafted a life-size statue of Dronacharya from clay and practiced diligently, imitating the master's teachings and techniques."

Saharsha's jaw dropped in astonishment. "Whoa, that's some serious dedication and creativity!"

Dad's eyes twinkled with admiration as he continued the tale. "Day and night, Ekalavya honed his skills, his fingers calloused from countless hours of pulling back the bowstring. The forest echoed with the rhythmic thrum of his arrows slicing through the air, each one finding its mark with unerring precision."

"Meanwhile, Dronacharya's royal students, though blessed with privilege and resources, struggled to match Ekalavya's unwavering commitment and natural talent."

Saumyaa's eyes widened in anticipation. "Did Dronacharya ever find out about Ekalavya's skill?"

Dad nodded solemnly. "One fateful day, as Dronacharya and his students were passing through the forest, they came across a barking dog, its mouth pierced by not one, but seven arrows – a feat of unparalleled marksmanship. Dronacharya immediately recognized the handiwork of a master archer and set out to find the source of such extraordinary skill."

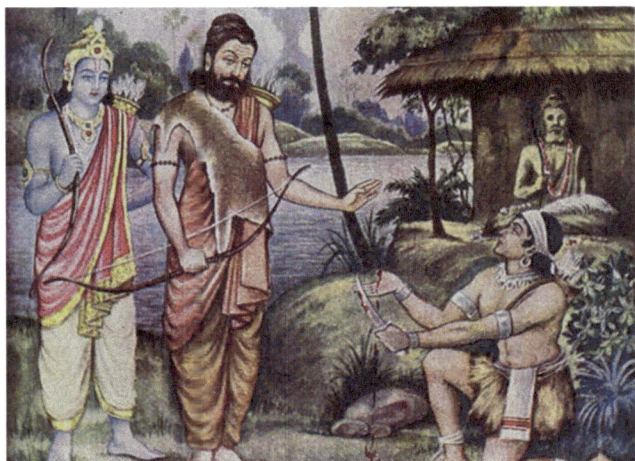

*(Ekalavya Cutting his thumb as a fee to Dronacharya)*

"To Dronacharya's astonishment, he discovered Ekalavya, a young boy from a humble background, who had surpassed even his most accomplished students through sheer determination and dedication."

Saharsha let out an awestruck whistle. "Incredible! What did Dronacharya do?"

Dad's expression grew contemplative, a reflection that mirrored Arjuna's own inner struggle. 'Dronacharya was torn,' he began, 'his rigid adherence to duty clashing with the undeniable potential before him. Ekalavya's story exemplifies the potential for greatness that lies within us all.'

Saumyaa beamed with delight. "See, Dad? Anyone can achieve greatness if they try hard enough and follow their passion!"

Dad smiles warmly at Saharsha and Saumyaa. "See, Saharsha and Saumyaa," he says, "these stories illustrate the concept of the soul in different ways. Ekalavya's story shows the potential for greatness that lies within each of us, regardless of background. The Tale of the Wise Old Sage explores the spiritual nature of the soul, that divine spark that connects us all."

Saharsha: "Cool! That makes it easier to understand," he exclaims.

Saumyaa: "Yeah, thanks Dad!" she adds.

Dad: "You're welcome!" Dad replies. "Now, the Bhagavad Gita offers its own perspective on the soul. It calls it the Atman, the true Self. This Atman is said to be eternal, unchanging, and the essence of who we truly are. It's like the puppeteer behind the physical body, the unchanging observer of our ever-changing thoughts and emotions."

Saharsha: "So the Atman is kind of like the driver of a car?"

Dad: "That's an interesting way to think about it, Saharsha! The car is our physical body, and the driver is the Atman, our true Self. The driver uses the car to navigate the world, but the driver itself is separate from the car."

Saumyaa: "So what happens to the Atman when the car, I mean our body, wears out?"

Dad: "The Bhagavad Gita teaches us that the Atman is not destroyed when the body dies. It simply moves on to another life, carrying the lessons learned in this one."

Saharsha: "Whoa, that sounds kind of scary," Saharsha says with wide eyes.

Dad: "It can be a bit overwhelming at first," Dad assures him. "But the idea is that each life is an opportunity for the Atman to learn and grow. By living a good life, filled with compassion and righteousness, we can ensure a better future for our Atman in the next life."

Saumyaa: "Is that why the Bhagavad Gita talks about doing your duty?"

Dad: "Exactly, Saumyaa! Fulfilling your dharma, your rightful duty in life, is a way to live a life of purpose that benefits not just yourself but also the world around you. This, in turn, helps the Atman on its journey of growth."

Saharsha: "So the Bhagavad Gita is kind of a guidebook for the soul?"

Dad: "In a way, it is, Saharsha! It offers wisdom on how to live a meaningful life that benefits both your physical self and your eternal Atman."

Saumyaa: "This is a lot to think about, Dad. Can we learn more about Dharma next time?"

Dad: "Absolutely, Saumyaa! Dharma is an important concept in the Bhagavad Gita and understanding it will help us unlock even more of the book's wisdom. Now, how about a glass of milk before bed?"

Saumyaa and Saharsha gazed at their dad, their eyes shining with newfound reverence for the profound wisdom hidden within the depths of their own souls. And from that day forward, they embarked on a journey of inner exploration, seeking to connect with the eternal Atman that resided within each of them.

## CHAPTER SUMMARY: THE YOGA OF WISDOM IN ACTION

This chapter of the Bhagavad Gita delves into the concept of the soul and performing actions without attachment to the fruits of those actions. Here are the key takeaways:

- **The Eternal Soul (Atman):** The chapter introduces the concept of the Atman, the true and eternal Self that resides within each person. It's compared to the unchanging driver of a car (the body).

- **The Cycle of Karma:** Our actions (karma) create consequences, both positive and negative, that influence our future lives.

- **Breaking Free from Karma:** By performing selfless actions and gaining knowledge of the Self (God), one can break free from the cycle of karma and rebirth.

- **Selfless Action vs. Desire-Driven Action:** The chapter emphasizes acting without being attached to the outcome. Doing your duty (dharma) for the sake of duty itself, rather than for personal gain, is considered the ideal way to act.

- **The Role of a Guru:** A true teacher or guru can guide us on the path of self-knowledge and help us understand complex spiritual concepts.

The chapter used stories like Ekalavya's dedication to archery to illustrate the potential for greatness within each person, and the Tale of the Wise Old Sage to explore the spiritual nature of the soul.

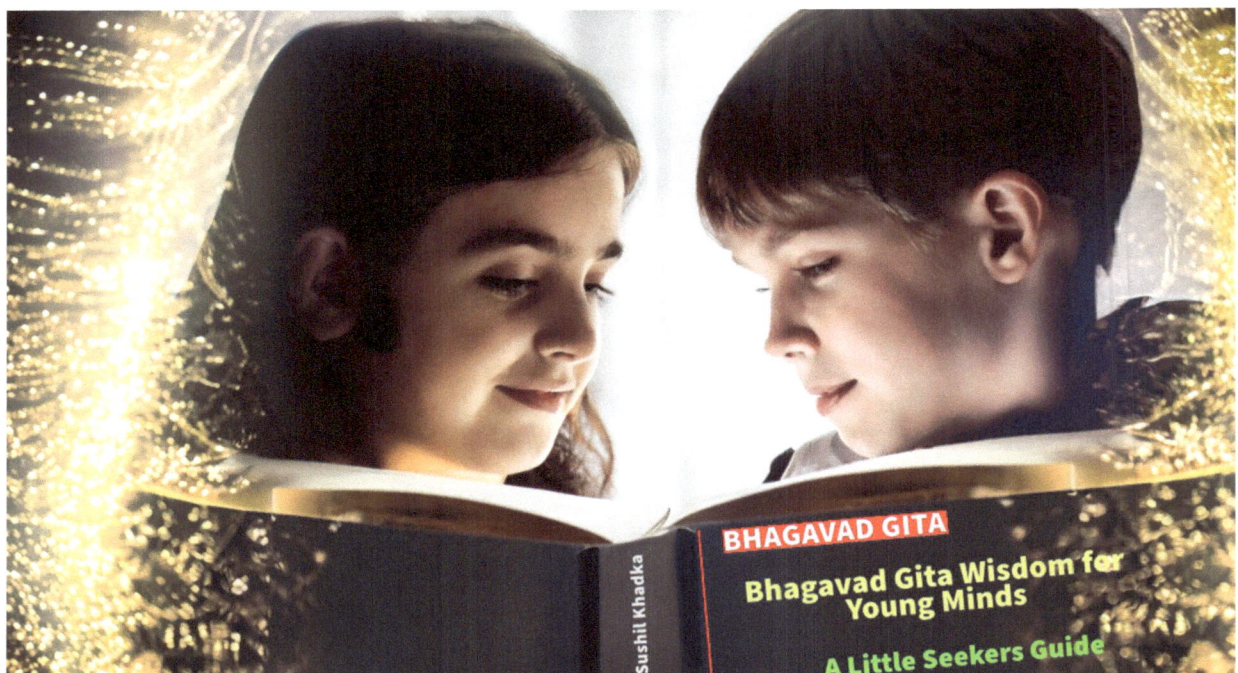

# Chapter 5: Doing Good Without Expecting Rewards

## Karma Yoga – The Path of Action Without Attachment

"

### *Ready to Be a Ripple Maker?*

*Saumyaa and Saharsha dive into the wondrous world of Karma Yoga The Bhagavad Gita teaches them the power of good deeds, no matter how small.*

*Plant a seed of kindness and watch it bloom into a more positive world!*

*Is helping a friend or sharing a smile enough? Discover the secret recipe for happiness and the joy of giving without expecting anything in return.*

*Chapter 5: Unleash the Karma Yogi within and watch your kindness ripple outward!*

Ready for an adventure, Saharsha, and Saumyaa? Dad's eyes sparkled like stars as he knelt down. Remember how Arjuna was stuck in a tough spot last time? Today, we meet the wise Krishna again, and he'll show us two secret paths to happiness!

Saharsha's eyes widened. **Two paths?** That's way cooler than finding buried treasure!

Saumyaa giggled. But Dad, giving up everything sounds scary, like being lost at sea without a compass.

Dad chuckled. Great point, Saumyaa! Here's the surprise: Krishna says there's an action path that's perfect for adventurers like you and Saharsha!

Action? Like fighting dragons? Saharsha perked up, picturing himself as a brave knight.

Not quite, Dad smiled. This path is called Karma Yoga, like being a superhero – but with a twist. You fight for what's right, but you don't care about winning medals or bragging.

I have a purpose for your pain, a reason for your struggle and a reward for your faithfulness, trust me and don't give up.

**BHAGAVAD GITA**

REWARD AHEAD

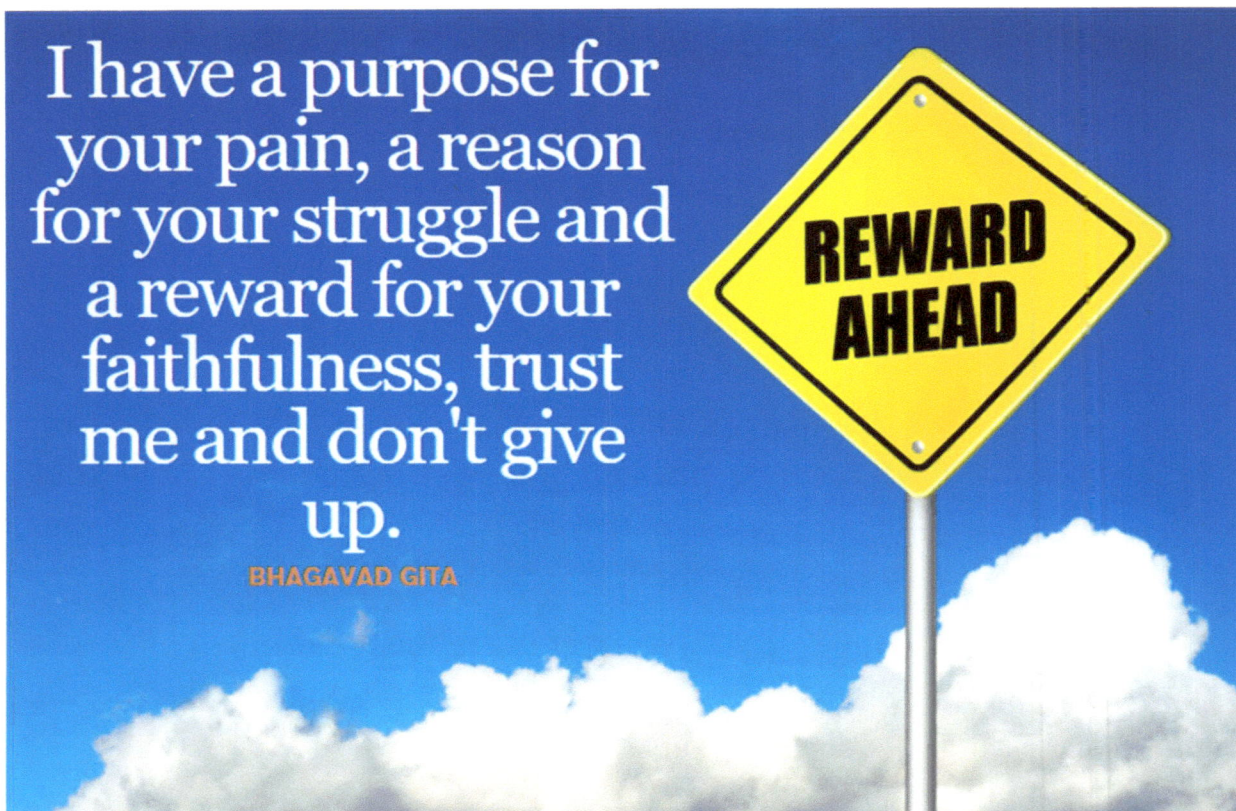

So, *it's like helping a friend win a game even if you don't get to hold the trophy?* Saumyaa asked thoughtfully.

Exactly! Dad said excitedly. Even small things you do to help others, because it's the right thing, become victories in Karma Yoga. Remember how we talked about karma last time?

Yeah, Saharsha chimed in, **good deeds lead to good things, and bad deeds lead to bad things,"** Saharsha finished, but his voice trailed off a little uncertainly.

Dad smiled warmly. "That's part of it, Saharsha. But Karma Yoga is a bit more than just rewards and punishments. It's about doing the right thing, even if it's hard, without getting attached to the outcome."

Saumyaa tilted her head. "So, even if you help someone and they don't say thank you, it still counts as good karma?"

"Exactly, Saumyaa!" Dad said, snapping his fingers. "It's about doing your duty, serving others selflessly, and focusing on the action itself, not the result."

Saharsha pondered this for a moment. "But what if someone's always mean to you, even though you try to be nice? Isn't that unfair?"

Dad nodded. "Life can be unfair sometimes, Saharsha. But Karma Yoga teaches us not to control others' actions, only our own. We can choose kindness even in the face of negativity. It might not change them, but it strengthens and purifies our own hearts."

Dad said, "In Karma Yoga, you do your duty, like a brave knight protecting his kingdom. But you don't wait for a pat on the back. You do it because it's the right thing to do."

Saumyaa tilted her head. What about the other path, Dad? The one where you leave everything behind?

That path, called renunciation, Dad explained, is like being a super-secret spy on a mission to solve a big mystery, just like Krishna talks about. It takes a lot of focus and bravery, just like a spy behind enemy lines.

Wait, Saharsha interrupted, can't a spy still help people, even if they don't know who's helping them?

Dad grinned. Amazing question, Saharsha! Krishna says some people can be secret spies for good, even while living normal lives. It's all about letting go of wanting things in return, like a spy who doesn't care about cool gadgets or fancy rewards, but just wants to complete the mission – to help others find peace and happiness."

Dad continued, "Let's talk about Karma Yoga again! Remember, it's not just about big acts of bravery. Sometimes, the smallest kindness can make a big difference."

Saharsha furrowed his brow. "Like what?"

Dad chuckled. "Imagine Maya, your classmate who always sits alone at lunch. What if you decided to offer her a spot at your table?"

Saumyaa's eyes widened. "But what if the other kids don't like it?"

Dad smiled. "It might be a little awkward at first. But Maya might feel happy to have someone to talk to. Who knows, maybe the other kids will join in too!"

Saharsha pondered this. "So, even if it's hard, we should still be kind?"

Dad nodded. "Exactly, Saharsha. Karma Yoga is about doing the right thing, even if it's uncomfortable. You might not get a prize or a thank you, but you'll be creating a more positive atmosphere for everyone. And that, in itself, is a reward."

Saumyaa tilted her head. "But what if Maya ends up being mean or doesn't want to be friends?"

Dad patted her shoulder. "That's okay, Saumyaa. We can't control other people's actions, only our own. But even if your offer isn't accepted right away, you've planted a seed of kindness. Maybe someday, it will blossom into a beautiful friendship."

"The Bhagavad Gita teaches us that when we act selflessly, good things tend to happen, even if not in the way we expect. And that's the power of Karma Yoga – doing good for the sake of good, without getting caught up in the results," Dad finished.

Dad smiled warmly. "Alright, Saumyaa and Saharsha, how are you feeling about Karma Yoga now? Does the idea of doing good deeds without expecting anything in return make more sense?"

Saumyaa's brow furrowed. "Maybe a little. But what if you do something nice and it doesn't seem to make a difference? Like Maya sitting alone at lunch today."

Dad nodded thoughtfully. "That's a great question, Saumyaa. You see, Karma Yoga isn't about immediate rewards. It's like planting a seed. You might not see a flower bloom right away, but with care and time, something beautiful can grow."

Saharsha chimed in, "So, even if Maya doesn't have anyone to play with at lunch today, helping someone else could still be good Karma Yoga? And what if no one sees you do the good deed? Does it still count?"

Dad chuckled. "Excellent question, Saharsha! As the proverb says, 'True charity is done anonymously.' In Karma Yoga, it's the act of doing good for the sake of good that matters, not the recognition."

Saumyaa chimed in, "So, even if you pick up someone's dropped pencil at school, even though no one saw you, it's still good Karma Yoga?"

Dad grinned. "Exactly, Saumyaa! Another proverb reminds us, 'Little strokes fell great oaks.' Every small act of kindness, no matter how seemingly insignificant, contributes to a positive world. It might be a small pebble you add to a pile, but eventually, it can make a big difference."

Saharsha pondered this for a moment. "But wouldn't it feel better if someone said thank you?"

Dad patted Saharsha's shoulder. "Feeling good about doing the right thing is definitely part of the reward, Saharsha. But Karma Yoga teaches us not to be attached to receiving something back. Remember, 'What goes around, comes around.' Your good deeds might not bring immediate results, but like a seed being nurtured, they have the potential to blossom into something positive, even if it's not in the way you expect."

Dad winked. "Think of yourself as a little Karma Yogi in training! You focus on doing the right thing, helping others without expecting anything in return, and the universe takes care of the rest. As another proverb says, 'The mill grinds slow, but sure.' Your good deeds, big or small, will eventually contribute to a happier world for yourself and those around you."

"So, even small acts are like the delicate flowers that add color and variety?" Saumyaa's eyes sparkled with understanding.

"Exactly, Saumyaa! And sometimes, a small act of kindness can have a ripple effect, leading to something much bigger.

Saharsha wasn't quite convinced yet. "But Dad, wouldn't people eventually stop being helpful if they never got thanked or rewarded?"

"That's a good point too, Saharsha," Dad said. "The thing is the reward in Karma Yoga isn't always something external. It's the good feeling you get from helping others, knowing you've made a positive difference in the world. It's a kind of inner peace and satisfaction that comes from doing the right thing."

Saumyaa pondered this for a moment. "So, it's like a superhero who gets a secret thrill from saving the day, even if no one knows who they are?"

Dad chuckled. "You could say that, Saumyaa! But in Karma Yoga, the reward is even greater because it's not just about yourself. It's about creating a more positive world for everyone."

Saharsha, still deep in thought, tapped his chin. "Dad, what if someone pretends to be nice and helpful, just to get a reward later? Is that still Karma Yoga?"

This question caught Dad by surprise. He hadn't considered that angle before. "Wow, Saharsha, that's a very insightful question! True Karma Yoga comes from a genuine desire to help, not from a place of expectation. It's like the difference between planting a seed because you want beautiful flowers or planting it because you expect someone to give you a prize for it."

Saumyaa, ever the curious one, piped up, "But Dad, if we can't see the future, how do we know if a good deed will lead to something good in return? What if we help someone, and it actually turns out bad?"

Dad smiled, impressed by their critical thinking. "That's a great question, Saumyaa! The truth is, we can't always control the outcome of our actions. But in Karma Yoga, the focus is on doing what you believe is right in the moment. Even if things don't turn out as expected, you can take comfort in knowing you acted with a good heart."

Saharsha, his eyes gleaming with curiosity, leaned forward. "So, Dad, is Karma Yoga like a secret code for happiness? Like if we follow all the rules, we're guaranteed to be happy?"

Dad chuckled. "There's no guaranteed path to happiness, Saharsha. But Karma Yoga certainly helps! It teaches us to focus on doing good for others, and that in itself brings a sense of joy and fulfillment. It's like a recipe with many ingredients – *kindness, selflessness, and a dash of acceptance* – that can lead to a happier life."

Saharsha and Saumyaa yawned, their eyelids growing heavy. The adventures of Karma Yoga had taken them on a journey filled with helpful heroes and unexpected rewards.

"Wow, Dad, ' Saumyaa mumbled, snuggling closer. "So many ways to be kind!"

"Exactly, Saumyaa," Dad whispered. "Remember, even small acts of kindness can make a big difference. And the good feeling you get from helping others? That's a reward all its own."

Saharsha's eyes fluttered shut. "Secret code for happiness..." he murmured, a sleepy smile playing on his lips.

Dad chuckled softly. "Maybe not a secret code, Saharsha," he said, tucking them both in. "But definitely a good recipe to try."

With thoughts of helping hands and hidden good deeds dancing in their dreams, Saharsha and Saumyaa drifted off to sleep, ready to face a new day filled with opportunities to practice Karma Yoga.

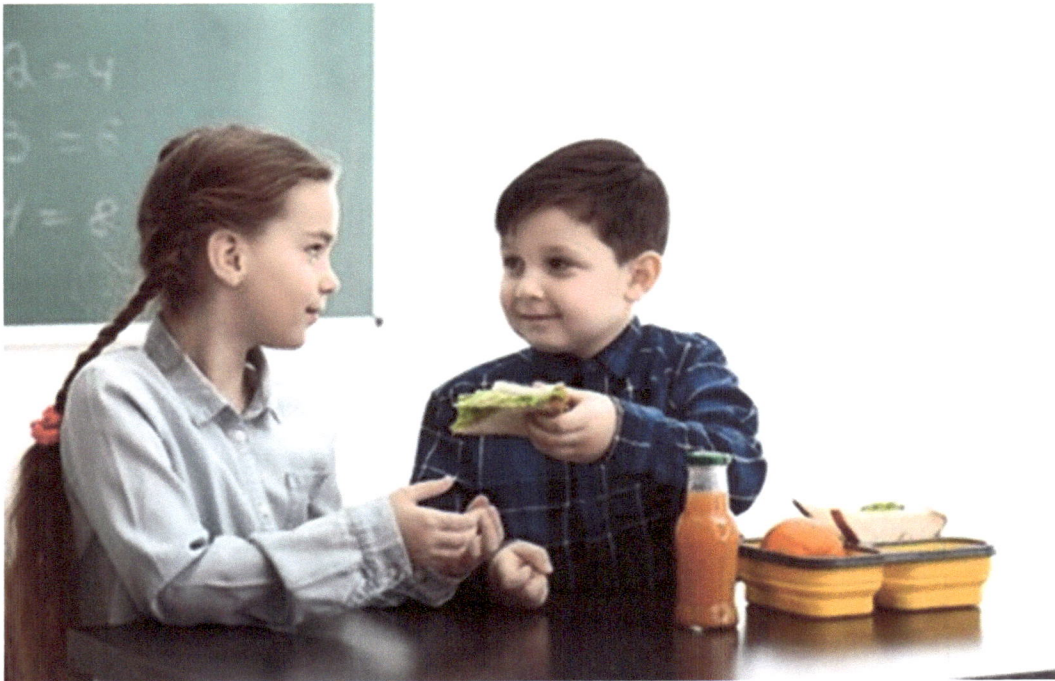

*Sharing food with a classmate less fortunate*

## CHAPTER SUMMARY: KARMA YOGA – THE PATH OF THE ACTION HERO

This chapter explores the concept of Karma Yoga from the Bhagavad Gita. Dad explains it to Saharsha and Saumyaa using engaging stories and relatable examples.

**Key Points:**

- Karma Yoga is a path of action focused on doing good deeds without expecting rewards.

- It's like being a superhero who fights for what's right but doesn't care about trophies or recognition.

- Even small acts of service, done with a kind heart, contribute to Karma Yoga.

- The reward in Karma Yoga is the inner peace and satisfaction that comes from helping others.

- True Karma Yoga comes from genuine desire to help, not from a place of expectation.

- Focusing on doing the right thing in the moment is key, even if the outcome is uncertain.

## Thought-provoking Questions:

- Are small acts of kindness enough, or are big heroic deeds more important? (Discussed through a garden analogy)

- Can someone pretend to be helpful for a reward and still practice Karma Yoga? (True Karma Yoga comes from genuine desire to help)

- What if a good deed leads to a bad outcome? (Focus is on doing what you believe is right in the moment)

- Is Karma Yoga a guaranteed path to happiness? (It promotes happiness through kindness and selflessness)

## Ending:

The chapter concludes with Saharsha and Saumyaa understanding the concept of Karma Yoga and feeling inspired to practice it in their own lives.

# Chapter 6: Finding Peace Inside – Exploring Meditation

> ## Ready to Embark on a Quest for Inner Peace?

*Saharsha and Saumyaa set off on a remarkable adventure. Finding Peace Inside! They discover a hidden power within themselves – meditation!*

*Is your mind ever like a bouncing monkey, full of restless thoughts? Learn how to calm your inner chatter and find stillness, just like our adventurous duo.*

*Uncover the ancient wisdom of the Bhagavad Gita and explore how meditation can unlock happiness and focus. Is it like mastering a cool bike trick? Join the journey and find out!*

The afternoon sun streamed through the window, casting playful squares of light onto the living room floor. Saharsha and Saumyaa burst through the door, their backpacks bouncing like overstuffed puppies and excited chatter tumbling out like a babbling brook.

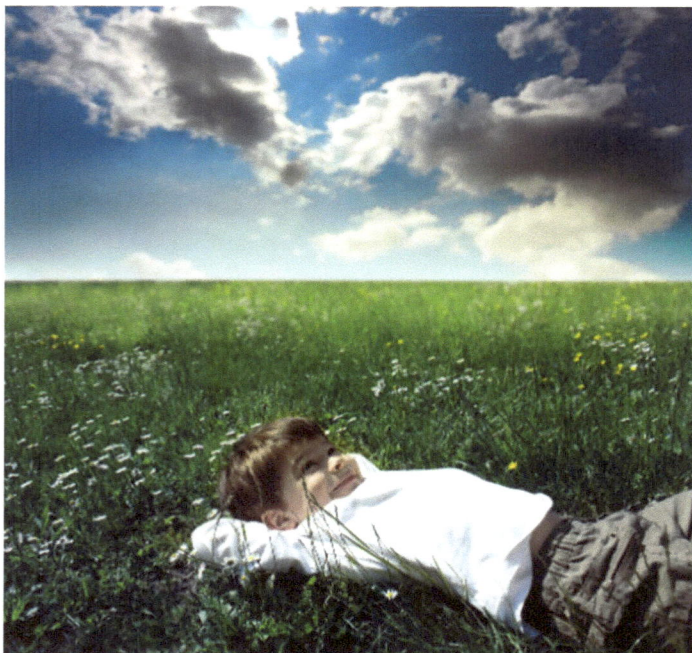

"Guess what happened at school today?" Saharsha yelled, barely catching his breath.

Saumyaa, ever the practical one, chimed in with a playful jab. "Yeah, Saharsha! Don't forget your apple slices, they'll give you the energy to tell the story right."

Saharsha, sheepishly grabbing his snack, slowed his pace a touch. "Okay, okay. You're right. School was...well, it was something else. But before I spill all the school beans, remember how Grandma mentioned different paths we can take in life? That made me think of something we learned about a while back, Dad. What was it called again... Karma Yoga?"

Tonight," Dad announced, a hint of intrigue in his voice, "we'll delve into the path of meditation, a secret superpower hidden within all of us! It's like the wisdom Lord Krishna shared in the Bhagavad Gita, remember? (Dad winks)

Saharsha, ever curious, tilted his head. "Lord Krishna? Did he have any cool quotes about this secret power?"

Dad chuckled. "He sure did, Saharsha! In fact, he even acknowledged how tough it can be to control your mind. Remember how sometimes you have trouble focusing in class, even though you want to? That's your mind being a little restless."

Saharsha and Saumyaa both nodded vigorously, a familiar struggle.

*"Lord Krishna said:*

*"Our minds can be like bouncy balls, always jumping around and making it hard to focus. When our minds are like that, it's difficult to find happiness or peace. But if we can learn to calm our minds and keep them still, it's like having a quiet friend to help us focus on good things."*

Saumyaa pondered this for a moment. "So, meditation helps us control our restless minds, kind of like how Karma Yoga helps us focus on doing good deeds without getting distracted by the outcome?"

Dad's eyes lit up. "Exactly, Saumyaa! Both Karma Yoga and meditation are about calming the mind and being present in the moment. When your mind is still, like a peaceful lake, it's easier to focus on doing good (Karma Yoga) or achieving inner peace (meditation). They go hand in hand, like two sides of the same coin."

"But even Lord Krishna knew it wouldn't be easy," Dad continued. "He also said:"

*'Even the smartest people can sometimes feel confused, like they have a mi'lion questions swirling in their heads. But if they practice calming their minds, maybe through yoga or just taking some quiet time, and remember something good, like a favorite song or a special person, they can start to feel steady and peaceful again.'"*

"Practice and yoga, huh?" Saharsha chimed in. "Sounds like something takes some work, just like mastering a new bike trick."

"Exactly, Saharsha!" Dad said, pulling them both closer. "At first, riding a bike felt wobbly, right? But with practice, you learned to balance. Meditation is similar. It might feel tricky at first, but with regular practice, you'll get better at calming your mind."

"There's an old saying: 'Practice makes perfect!' Meditation is kind of like learning a cool new trick on your bike. Even the calmest grown-ups, kind of like mind-bending masters, weren't always so good at quieting their minds. But with a little practice every day, just like you learned to balance without those training wheels, you'll get better at calming your thoughts too!"

"Can you tell us a story about practice making perfect?" Saumyaa's eyes sparkled with curiosity.

Dad grinned. *"Of course! Settle in, adventurers, and I'll tell you about a few tales that showcase the power of practice and meditation."*

## STORY 1: THE MONKEY AND THE STILL LAKE

Dad's voice got really interesting as he started to tell a story. "Once upon a time, there was a little monkey who lived in a big, green forest," he said. "This monkey loved to chase butterflies and swing on vines. He never stopped moving, and his mind was always thinking about something new."

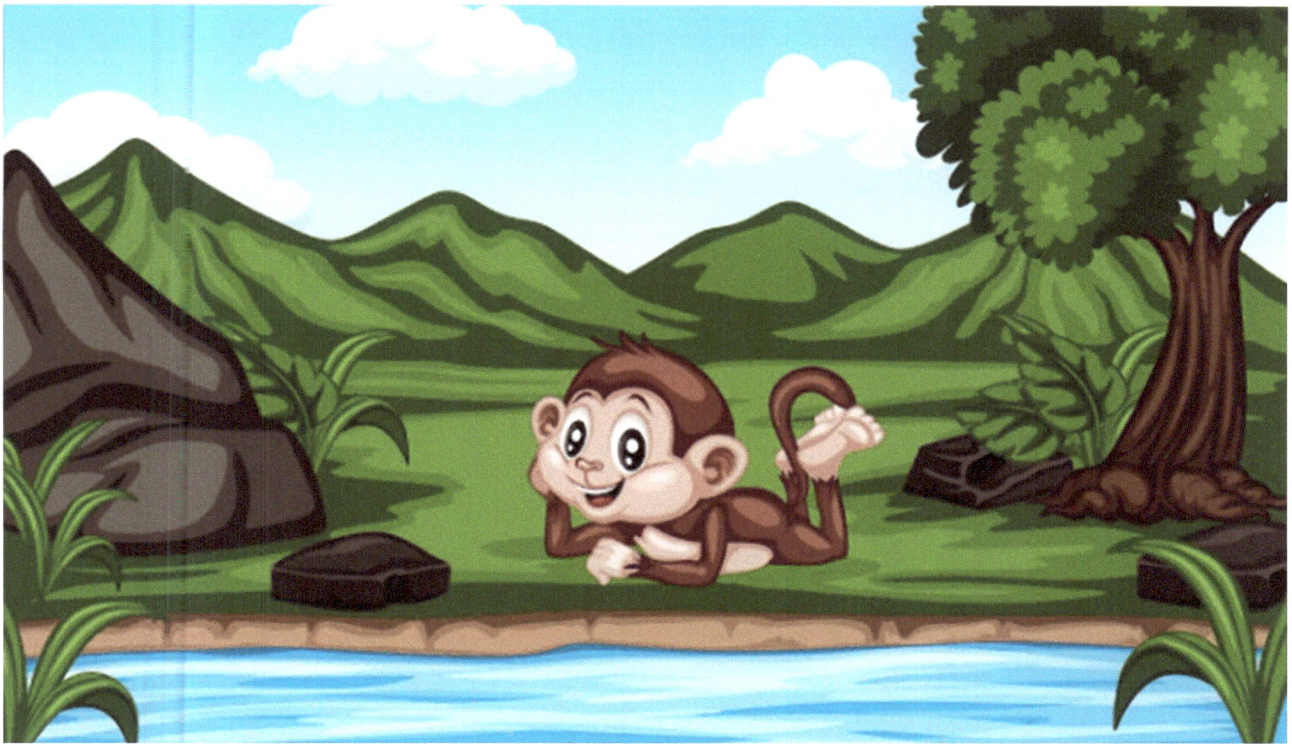

Saumyaa giggled. "He sounds like a busy bee!"

Dad grinned. "One sunny day, the monkey was hopping through the trees when he saw something amazing – a quiet pond! The water was so still, it looked like a mirror reflecting the big blue sky perfectly."

Curious, the monkey crept closer to get a better look. He was so excited that he forgot to be careful and dipped his paw right in the water! SPLASH! The smooth reflection broke into lots of little wiggles."

Saharsha gasped. "Aw, no! He ruined the beautiful reflection!"

"But the monkey didn't stop there," Dad said, shaking his head. "He splashed again and again, never allowing the waters to settle, forever disrupting the lake's serene state."

Saumyaa frowned. "Why would he keep doing that? Didn't he want to see the reflection?"

"Ah, that's an excellent question, Saumyaa," Dad replied. "You see, the monkey's mind was like a whirlwind, constantly jumping from one thought to another, never finding stillness or peace."

"That's when a wise old owl, perched on a nearby branch, hooted gently. 'Little one,' the owl said, 'why do you not simply sit and witness the beauty of the reflection? Only when the waters are undisturbed can you truly appreciate its majesty.'"

Saharsha nodded slowly, understanding dawning on his face. "So, the monkey had to learn to be patient and calm his mind, just like we do in meditation!"

Dad beamed. "Precisely, Saharsha! The monkey tried, but his restless thoughts kept disrupting the stillness of his mind. He realized he couldn't stop the thoughts completely, but the wise owl's words gave him an idea. He started observing his thoughts like clouds drifting across the sky. He didn't try to grab them or chase them away, just watched them pass by one by one. Slowly, his mind became calmer, like a clear blue sky after the clouds have moved on."

"And then?" Saumyaa asked, her eyes shining with anticipation.

"And then, my dear Saumyaa, the monkey finally saw the true beauty of the reflection – a perfect picture of the big blue sky in the still water, a sight of breathtaking wonder. Just like the calmness and clarity we can achieve through the practice of meditation."

Saharsha giggled. "So, our minds are mischievous monkeys?"

Dad chuckled, ruffling Saharsha's hair affectionately. "Sometimes, my son, our minds can indeed be as playful and restless as that little monkey. But meditation helps us train them to find stillness and focus, allowing us to truly appreciate the beauty and wonder all around us."

## STORY 2: DHRUVA, THE BOY WHO ACHIEVED PEACE

Dad's expression grew solemn as he began, "Let us travel back in time, where a young boy named Dhruva faced great unfairness and hardship."

Saumyaa's brow furrowed with concern. "What happened to him, Dad?"

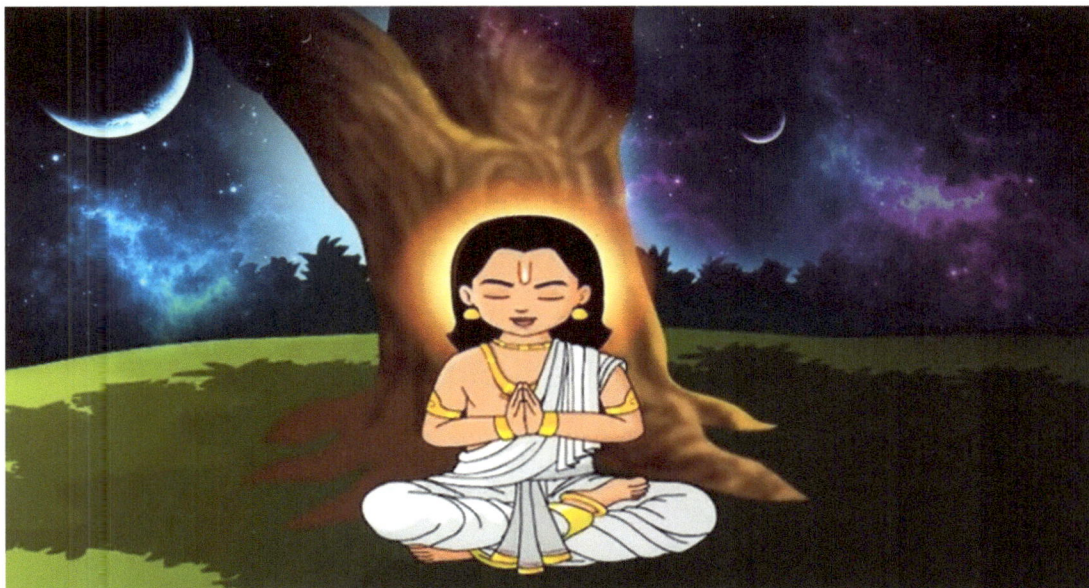

"Dhruva was the son of a king named **Uttānapāda**," Dad explained, and while the king loved Dhruva, the situation in the palace was complicated. Dhruva had a stepmother who had her own children. Unfortunately, this stepmother became jealous of Dhruva and favored her own sons. Despite the stepmother's actions, King Uttānapāda still cared for Dhruva, but the family dynamic created a challenging environment for him."

Saharsha shook his head sadly. "That's not right. Dhruva didn't deserve to be treated that way."

Dad nodded solemnly. "You're absolutely right, Saharsha. It's true, it wasn't fair. Feeling hurt and alone, Dhruva ran away from the palace. He wandered deep into the forest, tears streaming down his face. All he wanted was for his father to see him, to understand his pain. Lost and scared, Dhruva stumbled upon a quiet clearing bathed in moonlight. There, beneath the towering branches of an ancient tree, he sat down and poured his heart out. He cried and cried, calling out to his father, the king."

Saumyaa's eyes widened with curiosity. "So, Dhruva learned to meditate? Did it help him?"

"Indeed, it did, Saumyaa," Dad said, his voice filled with admiration. "In his darkest hour, Dhruva stumbled upon a wise sage who recognized the pain in his heart. The sage offered Dhruva a path to inner peace – meditation."

"Day and night, through scorching heat and bitter cold, Dhruva meditated with unwavering determination. He sat in quiet contemplation, the cool night air brushing against his skin, focusing his mind on the sound of his own breath. He let go of the hurt and anger that had consumed him, bit by bit, with each mindful breath."

"With unwavering determination, his goal remained clear – to find inner peace and strength."

Saharsha leaned forward, utterly captivated. "And then what happened, Dad?"

Dad's eyes twinkled with wonder. "Dhruva's dedication and perseverance were so remarkable that the supreme deity himself appeared before him in a blinding flash of light!

Saumyaa gasped, her hands flying to her mouth. "No way! That's incredible!"

Saharsha grinned from ear to ear. "Did Dhruva get an awesome reward, like superpowers or a magic sword?"

**Dad chuckled warmly. "An even greater reward, my son – something far more precious than any material possession." He paused for dramatic effect before continuing, "The deity granted Dhruva a state of ultimate happiness, peace, and self-realization. As a reward for his dedication, Lord Vishnu, the supreme Deity, transformed Dhruva into the Pole Star – the brightest star in the constellation Ursa Minor, forever serving as a symbol of perseverance and unwavering devotion.

Imagine Dhruva shining brightly in the night sky, a constant reminder of his journey."

Saumyaa's eyes shone with understanding. "So, through meditation, Dhruva found the true strength and peace within himself, didn't he?"

Dad nodded, beaming with pride. "That's exactly right, Saumyaa. Meditation isn't about gaining external rewards or superpowers. It's about unlocking the incredible potential, wisdom, and tranquility that already reside within each of us, just waiting to be discovered. It's like having a secret superpower inside you, waiting to be unleashed!"

Saharsha smiled contentedly. "That's pretty cool in its own way. I think I'd like to try meditating too!"

## CONNECTING THE STORIES AND INTRODUCING MEDITATION PRACTICE

Dad continued, skillfully weaving the stories together. "Just like the playful monkey learned to still his restless mind, and Dhruva achieved unwavering focus through meditation, there's another tale about a famous archer named Arjun."

Saharsha's eyes widened with interest. "Was Arjun a great warrior? Did he fight in epic battles?"

Dad nodded sagely. "Arjun was indeed a brave prince from a kingdom far, far away, who dreamt of becoming the greatest archer the land had ever seen. He practiced relentlessly, rising before dawn each day to perfect his aim."

"Just like the monkey practiced not splashing the water, right?" Saumyaa chimed in, making the connection.

"Precisely, Saumyaa!" Dad beamed. "Much like the determined monkey, Arjun trained diligently. He shot arrows at targets of all shapes and sizes, in all kinds of weather conditions. He learned from the wisest teachers, mastering techniques and strategies of archery."

Saharsha nodded, utterly engrossed in the tale. "But even with all that practice, I bet his mind sometimes got restless, just like the monkey's!"

Dad's eyes twinkled with admiration. "You're absolutely right, Saharsha. Despite Arjun's dedication, there were days when his arrows missed the mark, his mind flitting from thought to thought, like a butterfly chasing flowers in a meadow."

Saumyaa's brow furrowed in concern. "So, even with all that practice, Arjun couldn't control his mind?"

"Precisely, Saumyaa," Dad replied. "The frustration gnawed at him, making him question his abilities. One day, he encountered a wise old hermit renowned for his archery skills. The hermit watched Arjun practice, his keen eyes observing every move. Finally, the hermit spoke, his voice laced with gentle wisdom."

Dad paused for dramatic effect before continuing, "'Arjun,' the hermit said, 'your passion is admirable, but your mind is restless. It flits from thought to thought like a butterfly chasing flowers. True mastery comes not just from physical practice, but also from quieting the mind.'"

Saharsha's eyes widened with realization. "So, even with all that practice, his mind was still like an unruly monkey?"

Dad chuckled warmly. "In a way, yes, Saharsha! The hermit then shared a secret technique – meditation. He taught Arjun to sit still, close his eyes, and focus on his breath, letting go of all other thoughts. With regular practice, just like the monkey slowly learned to be still, Arjun discovered the power of a calm mind. His aim became unwavering, his focus laser sharp. He finally understood that mastering archery wasn't just about strength and technique but also about inner peace."

Saumyaa's eyes sparkled with understanding. "So, meditation helped both Arjun and the monkey to focus better and achieve their goals?"

Dad nodded, his expression filled with pride. "Absolutely, Saumyaa! Just like Arjun, the monkey, and Dhruva, with regular practice, meditation can help all of us tame our restless minds, making us calmer, happier, and more focused in everything we do, from school to hobbies and beyond."

Saharsha grinned eagerly. "Dad, can you teach us how to meditate too? I want to be as focused as Arjun and the monkey when they finally got it!"

Dad smiled warmly. "Of course, Saharsha! Meditation is a practice anyone can learn, even young adventurers like you and Saumyaa. It's all about training your mind to be a little calmer, just like the monkey learning to still the water. The first step is to find a quiet place, maybe on your bed or a comfy rug. Then, you can close your eyes gently and choose a special word or phrase, like 'peace' or 'calm,' to repeat silently in your mind. Each time you breathe in, think that word, and each time you breathe out, let go of any worries or distractions."

"As you focus on your word," Dad continued, "you might notice your mind wandering, like a playful puppy chasing butterflies. That's okay! When that happens, just gently bring your attention back to your word and your breath. The more you practice, the easier it will become to quiet your mind and find that inner peace."

## THE INVITATION TO PRACTICE

"The best part?" Dad said, his voice filled with excitement. "Since tomorrow is Saturday, and you won't have school to worry about, we can actually try a short meditation session together! How does that sound?"

Saharsha's initial enthusiasm seemed to wane a little. "Meditation? But won't it be boring?"

Dad anticipated this reaction. "Not at all, Saharsha! Think of it as an adventure for your mind. We can find a quiet spot, close our eyes, and focus on our breath, just like Arjun. It might feel strange at first, but with a little practice, it can be quite peaceful."

Saumyaa, ever the eager one, bounced in her seat. "I'm in! Can we start now?"

Dad chuckled. "Hold on there, Saumyaa! Let's grab some comfy cushions and find a quiet corner in the house. Then, I'll guide you both through a simple meditation session."

The prospect of an adventure for their minds, along with the promise of comfy cushions, piqued Saharsha and **Saumyaa's** curiosity. With a newfound openness, they were ready to embark on their first meditation journey, eager to see if they could tame their monkey minds and discover the inner peace found in stillness.

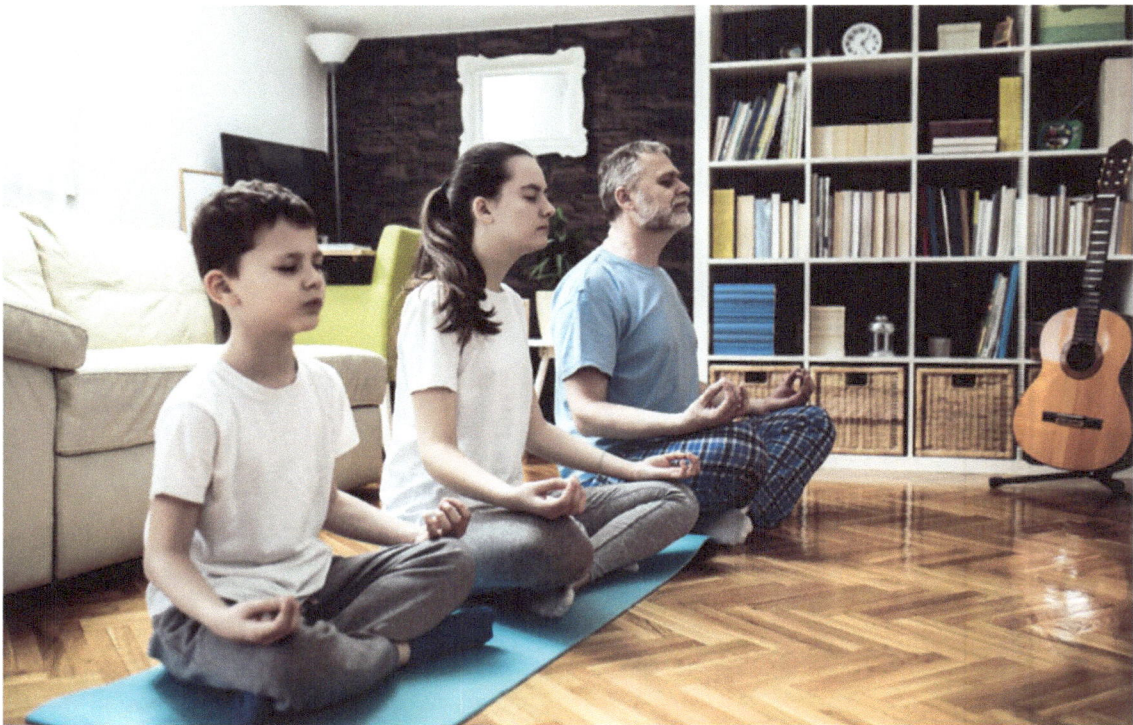

## CHAPTER SUMMARY: FINDING PEACE INSIDE

Saharsha and Saumyaa return from school, excited to share their day with Dad. Dad surprises them by proposing a new learning journey about meditation, a hidden "superpower" within all of us. He uses quotes from the Bhagavad Gita, a sacred Hindu scripture, to explain how a restless mind hinders focus and happiness.

The chapter uses three stories to illustrate the importance of practice and focus:

- **The Monkey and the Still Lake:** A playful monkey learns to quiet his mind to see the reflection in a lake, symbolizing the need to calm our thoughts for inner peace. (Saharsha asks a question about the monkey mind)

- **Dhruva, the Boy Who Achieved Peace:** Through meditation and unwavering focus, Dhruva attains inner peace despite facing challenges. (Saharsha asks about the reward, highlighting the focus on inner strength)

The chapter connects these stories to the concept of meditation, which Arjun, a skilled archer, uses to improve his focus and achieve mastery. (Saharsha and Saumyaa ask questions about the difficulty of controlling the mind)

Dad proposes a practical experience: a meditation session on Saturday, sparking curiosity and excitement in both Saharsha and Saumyaa despite their initial reservations.

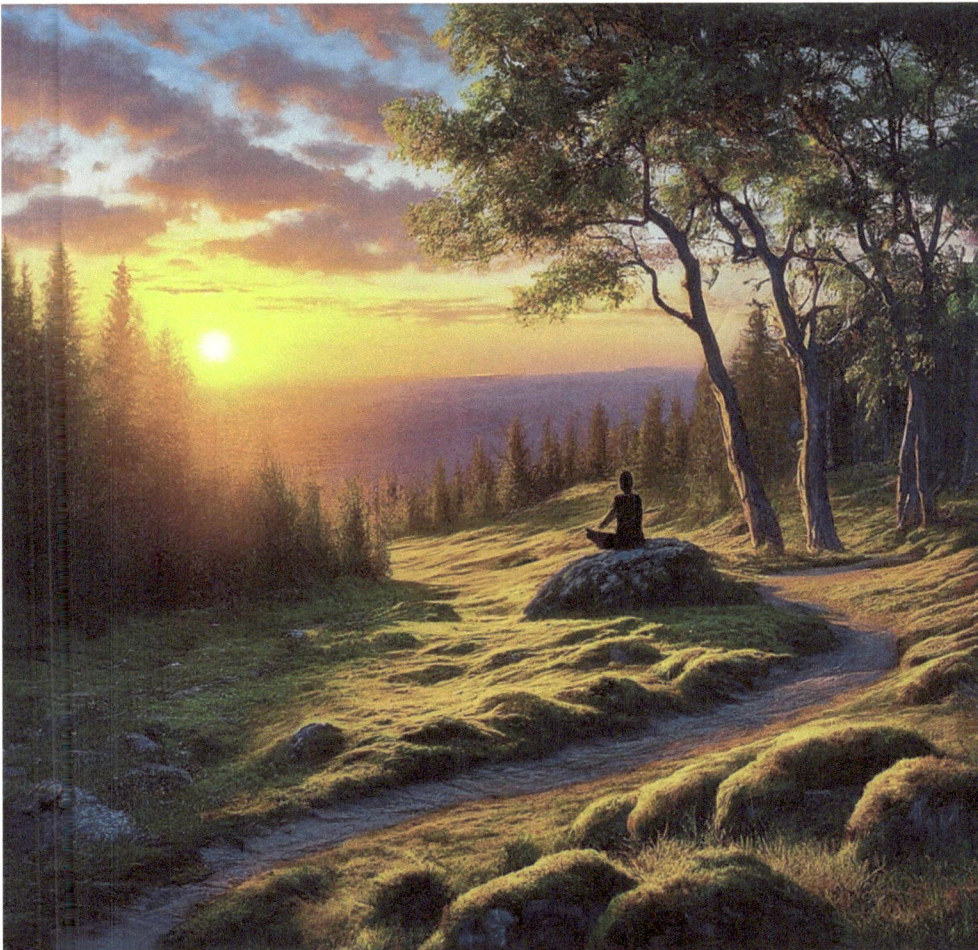

# Chapter 7: Learning About the World

## The Treasure Within

*A World Unfolds! Chapter 7: The Exploration Begins!*

*The library doors creak open, a world of knowledge waiting inside. Saumyaa and Saharsha, eyes sparkling with curiosity, grab dusty tomes on faraway lands. What secrets lie hidden on a spinning globe? Will they climb the tallest mountains or sail across vast oceans? Join the adventure! Explore bustling cities, marvel at ancient wonders, and uncover the breathtaking beauty of our planet. Chapter 7: Unleash your inner explorer! The world awaits!*

Saharsha and Saumyaa burst through the door, backpacks slung carelessly on their shoulders. Their excited chatter filled the room, a whirlwind of schoolyard adventures and classroom discoveries.

Dad looked up from his book, a warm smile spreading across his face. "Welcome back, explorers! What treasures did you unearth today?"

Saumyaa, ever the meticulous one, launched into a detailed explanation of a fascinating science experiment about plant growth. Saharsha, brimming with boundless energy, followed with a hilarious account of a near-disaster during dodgeball practice.

As their energy subsided, Dad leaned closer, his voice dropping to a conspiratorial whisper. " Today, we're going to explore treasure!" he said, his eyes twinkling with excitement. "But it isn't about pirates or buried gold! It's about finding a different kind of treasure – one hidden deep inside each of you!""

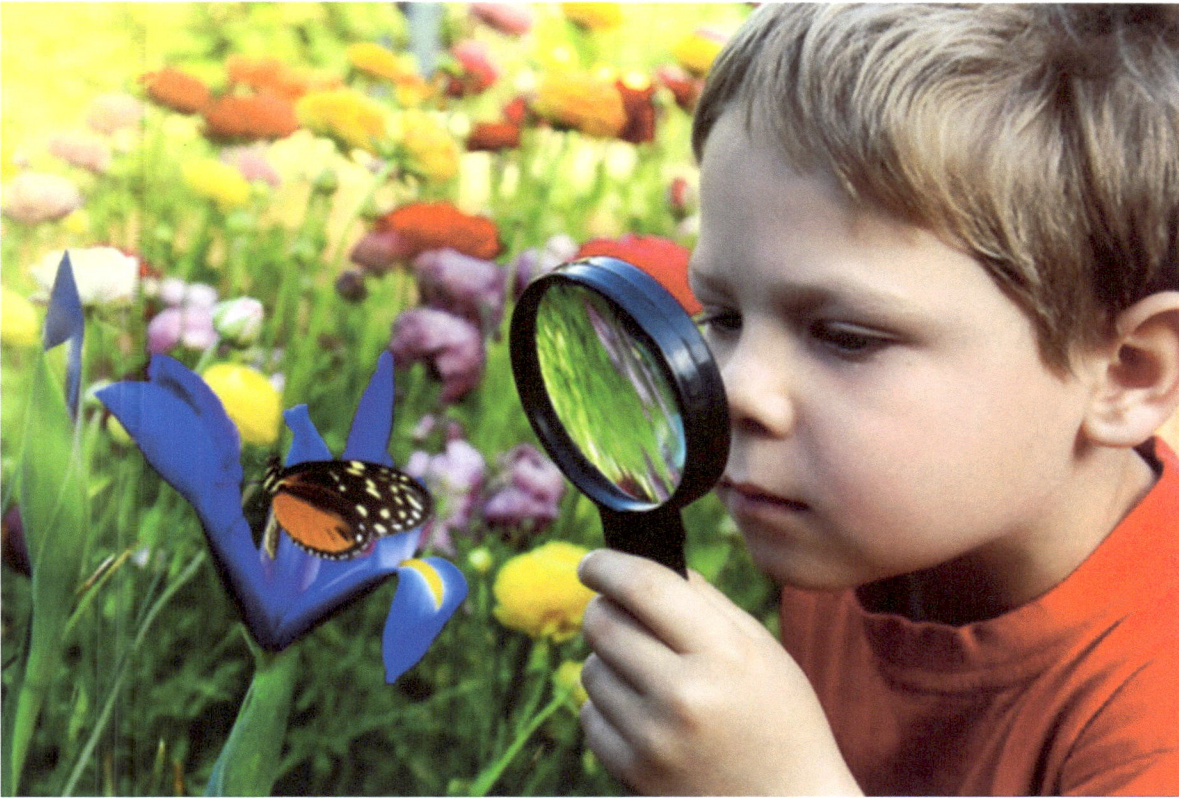

Saharsha's brow furrowed. "A treasure chest inside us? What kind of treasure are we talking about, Dad? Gold coins and jewels?"

Dad chuckled. "Not exactly, Saharsha! This treasure chest holds something even more valuable – self-knowledge. It's about understanding who you are, your strengths, weaknesses, and all the amazing things that make you unique!"

Saumyaa pondered this for a moment. "So, self-knowledge is like a map that helps us navigate ourselves?"

"Exactly, Saumyaa! It's like having a map that shows your hidden talents, helps you overcome challenges, and guides you towards your dreams."

"But how do we find this map, Dad?" Saharsha asked, his curiosity piqued.

"There are many ways, Saharsha," Dad replied. "Remember the stories we heard about the monkey calming his mind and Dhruva finding inner peace? Meditation is a tool that can help us unlock that same treasure within ourselves." *"Meditation is one powerful tool. It helps us quiet the constant chatter in our minds, like a noisy crowd at a marketplace, and allows us to see ourselves more clearly."*

Suddenly, a new question popped into Saharsha's head. "But wait, Dad," he interrupted, his brow furrowed in concentration. **"If we're all looking for this treasure within ourselves, who created the world outside of us?** Was it a giant treasure keeper who hid all these treasures?"

Dad smiled, his eyes twinkling with amusement. "That's a great question, Saharsha! Many people throughout history have wondered about the creation of the universe. There are many beliefs, but some believe in a single divine power, a creator of everything."

"So, there's just one God?" Saumyaa asked, tilting her head thoughtfully.

"Some religions believe in one God, while others believe in many gods and goddesses," Dad explained. "In Hinduism, for example, we have many deities like Ganesha, Shiva, Hanuman – all representing different aspects of the one divine power. It's like having a giant diamond with many beautiful facets – each facet reflecting a different quality of the same divine light." 'As an old proverb says, 'We are all like diamonds in the rough – with the potential for incredible beauty and brilliance waiting to be discovered.'"

"So, even though we pray to different deities, we're ultimately connecting with the same source?" Saumyaa's eyes widened with realization.

Dad nodded. "That's a way to understand it, Saumyaa. Meditation can help you connect with that inner source, the treasure chest of self-knowledge within, regardless of the form you choose to worship."

Saharsha: But Dad, can God take different forms?

Dad: Indeed, Saharsha. *God can manifest Himself in various forms, both seen and unseen. While some believe God is formless, others see Him in everything around us.*

Saumyaa: Dad, can you tell us a story that relates to this idea?

Dad: Of course! Let me tell you the story of the disciple and the mad elephant.

Once upon a time, in a village nestled within a dense forest, there lived a holy man (Guruji) who had many disciples. He taught them to see God in all beings and to bow down before them. One day, a disciple ventured into the forest to gather wood for the fire. Suddenly, he heard a shout.

"Get out of the way! A mad elephant is coming!"

Everyone except the disciple ran away in fear. However, he saw the elephant as God in another form. Why should he flee from God? He stood still, bowed before the elephant, and began meditating on God in the form of the elephant.

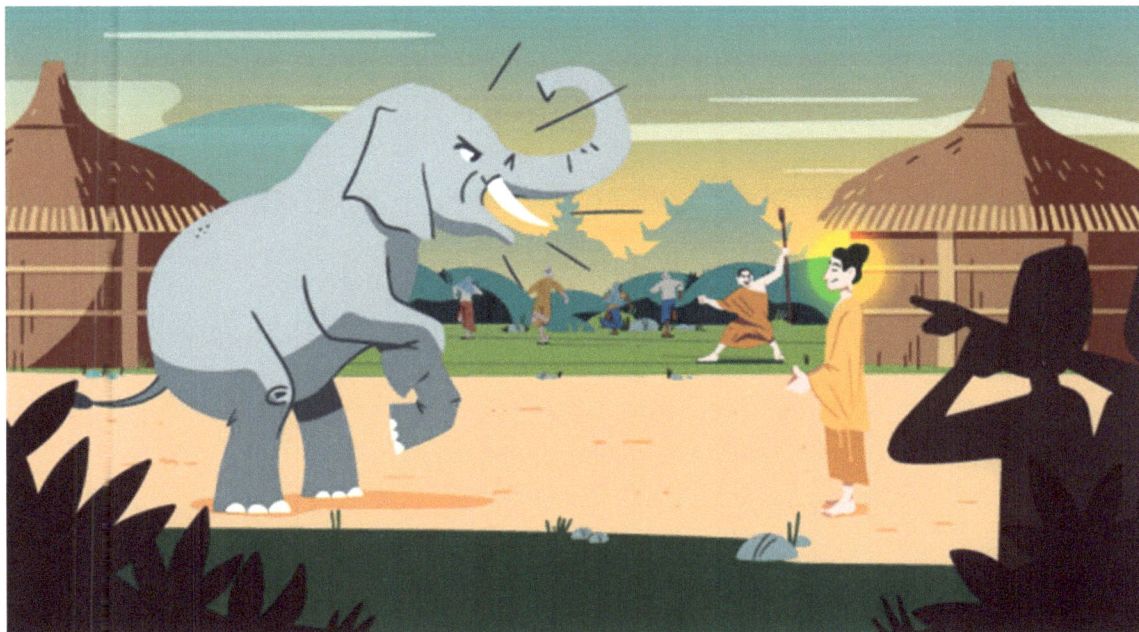

The mahout, or the elephant's trainer, shouted, "Run away! Run away!"

The disciple stood still, remembering his teacher's words - God is in everything! Even a grumpy elephant! So, when the elephant ran towards him, the disciple didn't move. He bowed low, greeting the "elephant-god."

The elephant, angry and huge, didn't care about the disciple's thoughts. It grabbed him with its trunk and threw him aside before continuing on its way.

The disciple, feeling dizzy and hurt, saw his worried fellow disciples around him. One asked, "Why didn't you run when you saw the elephant?"

Still feeling confused, the disciple rubbed his head and said, "Ouch! he exclaimed. Maybe some forms of gods give better blessings than others." he mumbled sheepishly.

The guruji smiled kindly. "You're right, my child," he said softly. "The elephant was like a god, but the mahout, who warned you, was also a form of divinity. He tried to keep you safe. You should have heeded his call. Remember, not everyone understands the divine in all things, and not all creatures know how to be kind and gentle yet, even though there's goodness inside them."

Saharsha: Wow, that's a great story, Dad! It really helps us understand how to see God in everything around us.

Dad: Exactly, Saharsha. The world is full of opportunities to connect with the divine. We just need to open our hearts and minds to see it.

Saumyaa: Thanks for sharing, Dad. It makes me feel closer to God knowing that He's always around us.

Dad smiled. "Now, are you both ready to begin your own journey inward, to discover the treasure chest of self-knowledge within yourselves?"

Saharsha and Saumyaa, their eyes wide with newfound wonder, exchanged excited glances. "Absolutely, Dad!" they chorused in unison.

Dad chuckled and guided them to gather some comfy cushions. They found a quiet corner in the house, settling themselves comfortably.

"Meditation can feel strange at first," Dad explained, his voice calming and soothing. "But with a little practice, it can become a powerful tool for self-discovery. Today, we'll start with a simple breathing exercise. Close your eyes and focus on your breath as it enters and leaves your body. Imagine your breath is like a gentle wave, washing over you and calming your mind."

Saharsha and Saumyaa closed their eyes, their initial giggles subsiding as they focused on their breath. The room fell silent except for the soft sound of their inhalations and exhalations.

After a few minutes, Dad's voice gently guided them back to the present moment.

"How was that, adventurers?" Dad asked with a warm smile.

Saharsha, his eyes still closed, spoke softly. "It felt weird at first, Dad, but kind of peaceful too."

Saumyaa nodded in agreement. "My mind was still a little like a busy bee, but it felt good to focus on something calm."

"That's a great start!" Dad said encouragingly. "Remember, meditation is a practice, like learning a new skill. The more you practice, the easier it becomes to quiet your mind and connect with yourself."

Saharsha: Dad, do you think this self-knowledge journey can help us discover our purpose in life? Like, why are we here?

Dad: That's a wonderful question, Saharsha! Self-knowledge is a key part of finding your purpose. As you learn more about your strengths, interests, and values, you'll start to see what lights you up and what kind of impact you want to make on the world.

Saumyaa: Can meditation help us become kinder people, Dad? Maybe help us understand others better?

Dad: Absolutely, Saumyaa! When you're calm and focused, you're better able to see things from other people's perspectives. Meditation can help you develop compassion and understanding for yourself and others.

Saharsha: So, the more we explore this treasure chest within ourselves, the more we can unlock all sorts of amazing things?

Dad: Exactly, Saharsha! Self-knowledge is a lifelong journey, full of exciting discoveries. It's like a treasure map that keeps unfolding, revealing new paths and possibilities as you go.

With a newfound sense of possibility, Saharsha and Saumyaa were eager to continue their exploration of the world within. They knew their journey towards self-knowledge had just begun, filled with the promise of exciting discoveries and a deeper understanding of themselves, the divine around them, and their place in the world.

## CHAPTER SUMMARY: THE TREASURE WITHIN

Saharsha and Saumyaa return home excited to share their day's adventures. Their father suggests a different kind of adventure - a journey inwards to discover the "treasure chest" within each of them, symbolizing self-knowledge.

This self-knowledge is like a map that helps them understand their strengths, weaknesses, and unique qualities. Meditation is introduced as a tool to quiet the mind and gain clarity. Saharsha questions the origin of the world, prompting a discussion about the divine.

Their father explains that some believe in a single God, while others believe in many gods and goddesses representing different aspects of one divine power. He uses the analogy of a giant diamond with many facets to illustrate this concept.

Saharsha asks if God can take different forms, leading to the story of the disciple and the mad elephant. This story highlights the importance of discernment and listening to inner guidance alongside recognizing the divine in all beings.

Feeling closer to God knowing He's present everywhere, Saharsha and Saumyaa are ready to begin their meditation practice. They find the experience calming despite initial challenges.

The chapter concludes with Dad encouraging them to see meditation as a practice, like learning a new skill. Thought-provoking questions are added to spark further exploration:

- Saharsha ponders if self-knowledge can help them discover their life's purpose.

- Saumyaa wonders if meditation can foster kindness and understanding.

- Saharsha reflects on the potential for self-discovery and unlocking their inner treasures.

The chapter ends with a sense of possibility as Saharsha and Saumyaa embark on their journey of self-knowledge, understanding the divine, and finding their place in the world.

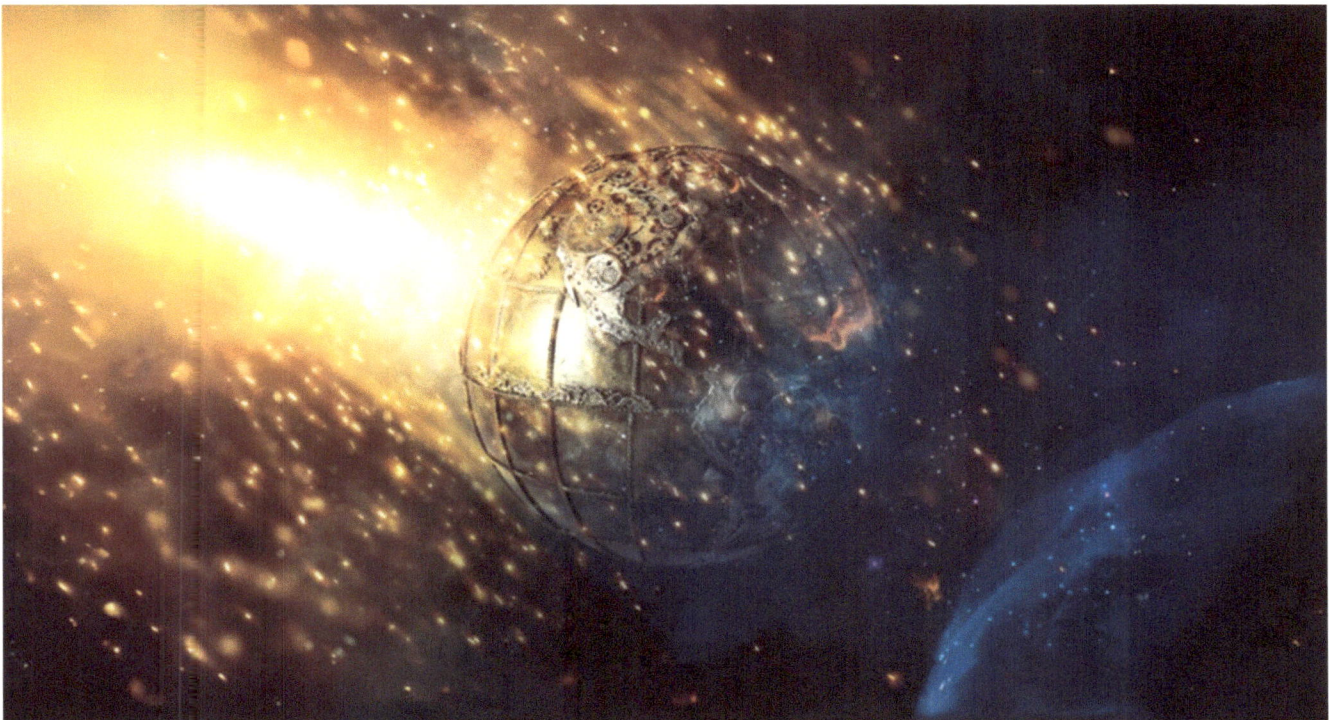

# Chapter 8: Believing in Something Bigger

## A Journey of Questions and Discovery

"

### *Awe-Inspiring Questions! Chapter 8: The Big Why*

*Crimson dust settles on a battlefield, the echoes of war fading. Arjuna, weary but resolute, looks up at the vast night sky. Millions of stars shimmer, each a silent question mark.*
*What is our place in this grand universe? Are we alone? Why are we here?*
*Saumyaa and Saharsha embark on a quest unlike any other: a journey of wonder and curiosity. They delve into diverse beliefs, explore the universe's mysteries, and grapple with life's biggest questions.*
*Chapter 8: Unleash Your Inner Wonderer! Explore the mysteries of existence!*

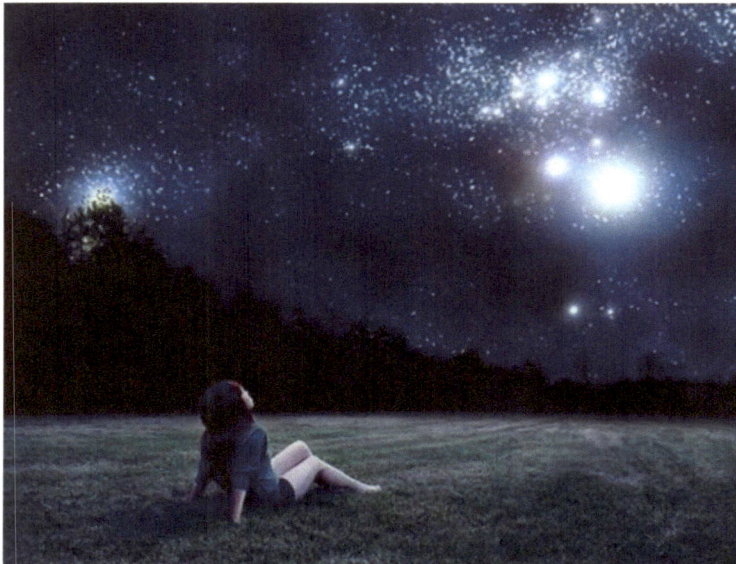

Saumyaa, Saharsha, and their Dad were curled up together on the comfy rug, bathed in the warm glow of the evening lamp. The day's hustle and bustle had settled, replaced by a quiet curiosity that crackled in the air.

*"Dad,"* Saumyaa began, her brow furrowed in concentration, "at the temple today, I heard something about Brahma.

But everyone seems to use different words — Brahma, Brahman, even Brahma with a capital B. It's all so confusing!"

Saharsha, ever the eager listener, chimed in, "Yeah, and what about Karma? Is it just about doing good deeds, or is there more to it?"

Dad smiled, his eyes twinkling with amusement. **"Those are fantastic questions, my adventurers!** The world of spirituality can be a vast ocean, filled with fascinating concepts and sometimes confusing terms. But fear not, we can explore it together, one question at a time."

He settled himself comfortably and began, *Have you ever seen a beautiful carpet, with all sorts of patterns and colors woven together? Imagine the entire universe is like that, but way, way bigger! Brahma, with a big B, is the master weaver who made it all. He's like the artist who started the whole picture!*

Saumyaa's eyes widened. "So, Brahma is like a giant artist, painting the stars and shaping the planets?"

Dad chuckled. "In a way, yes! But Brahma is also something more. There's another concept, Brahma with a lowercase b, or Brahman. This refers to the universal spirit, the essence that flows through all living things. It's like the invisible thread that binds everything together in the tapestry."

Saharsha scratched his head. "So, there's a creator Brahma and a universal spirit Brahma? Are they the same?"

Dad nodded. "Think of it like a coin. Brahma, the creator, is one side, while the universal spirit is the other. They are two aspects of the same divine reality."

Saumyaa pondered this for a moment. "But Grandma always says there's one supreme God. Does that fit in somehow?"

"Absolutely!" Dad said, his voice filled with excitement. "Many people in Hindu religion believe in this supreme being, called Para Brahman or Paramātmā. It's like the source of all creation, the ultimate light from which everything else flows, including Brahma, the creator, and the universal spirit, Brahman."

"Whoa," Saharsha breathed, his imagination ignited. "So, it's like a giant chain of light, with the supreme God at the top and Brahma and Brahman connected below?"

Dad smiled. "A beautiful analogy, Saharsha! Now, Karma isn't just about doing good deeds. It's the **law of cause and effect**, the principle that every action has a reaction. The choices we make, good or bad, create a ripple effect that influences our future."

Saumyaa tilted her head. "So, if I help an old lady cross the street, that's good Karma, right?"

"Exactly, Saumyaa! But Karma is more than just good and bad deeds. It's also about learning from our experiences and evolving as souls."

Suddenly, Saharsha's eyes sparkled with a new question. "Dad, what happens after we die? Do we just... disappear?"

Dad's voice softened. "The idea of being reborn after we die is a belief held by many religions, not just Hindus. It's called reincarnation, the cycle of birth, death, and rebirth. In some religions, people believe our good and bad deeds, kind of like a scorecard, influence what we come back as in the next life. Our Karma determines our next life form. We could be reborn as humans again, or maybe even an animal."

Saumyaa shivered. "Being reborn as a snake doesn't sound very pleasant! '

Dad chuckled. "That's why it's important to strive for good Karma, to live a life that helps us evolve towards a higher state of being."

"But is there a way to escape this cycle of rebirth?" Saharsha asked, his voice filled with curiosity.

Dad smiled. "That's where the concept of **Moksha, or liberation**, comes in. Imagine life is like a big game with many levels. Moksha is like reaching the final top level, where you've learned everything there is to learn and can finally be at peace. It's like an old saying, **'True happiness isn't found in having things, but in who you are.'** When we achieve true self-realization, when we understand the good and light that shines within ourselves, we break free from the cycle of wanting more and more things. It's like a butterfly trapped in a cocoon. It's comfy and safe inside, but the butterfly can't truly fly or experience the beauty of the world. Moksha is like the butterfly breaking free from the cocoon, finally able to experience all that life has to offer."

Saumyaa's eyes shone with understanding. "So, when we break free from wanting too much and find that special light inside, that's Moksha, right?"

Dad nodded. "Exactly, Saumyaa! It's like a beautiful flower blooming. The more we nurture the good within ourselves, the brighter our inner light shines. There are many paths to Moksha, Saumyaa. Meditation, following your Dharma (life purpose), and acts of service are all ways to connect with the divine and work towards liberation."

Saharsha tilted his head. **"Dharma? What's that?"**

Dad chuckled. "Dharma is a bit like a special map guiding you through your life. It's about understanding your unique talents and using them to make the world a better place. Maybe you're good at helping others, or maybe you love creating art. Your Dharma is your way of sharing your light with the world."

Saumyaa's brow furrowed in thought. "So, finding Moksha is about being kind, using your talents, and letting your inner light shine?"

Dad beamed. "You've got it, Saumyaa! It's a beautiful journey of self-discovery, and we can all embark on it together. Remember, even the smallest acts of kindness can light up the world."

Dad tucked Saharsha and Saumyaa into bed, the night buzzing with the echoes of their conversation.

"One last story before you drift off," Dad said with a smile. "This one is about a great king named Bharata. He was wise and just, ruling his kingdom with a steady hand. But even the wisest can struggle with attachment. One day, King Bharata became very fond of a beautiful deer he found in the forest. He spent all his time playing with it, forgetting about his duties as king. This wasn't good for the kingdom, and it made Bharata sad too."

Saharsha's brow furrowed. "So, spending too much time with something you love can be bad?"

Dad smiled. "That's a great question! This story teaches us that even good things can become a problem if we get too attached to them. It's important to remember that there are many things to love and care for in the world. *Finding true happiness means being aware of yourself and not getting too hung up on things you can't control.*"

Saumyaa yawned, her eyelids drooping. "So even kings have to learn to let go?"

"Everyone does, Saumyaa," Dad replied gently. "Letting go can be the hardest thing, even for the strongest of us. We talked about the vastness of the universe, the wisdom hidden within ourselves, and the importance of letting go of things that no longer serve us. These are all pieces of the grand puzzle, our own unique journey of self-discovery."

With that, Dad kissed them goodnight. Sleep washed over them, filling their dreams with galaxies, heroes (removed as not mentioned earlier), and the quiet spark within. The vastness felt overwhelming yet comforting, promising adventures to come.

The next morning, Saumyaa found Dad reading in the kitchen. "Dad," she whispered, "can we learn more about meditation? Maybe it can help us find that light within."

Dad smiled. "Excellent idea! Meditation calms the mind and connects you with yourself. It's not easy, but practice brings peace and clarity."

Saharsha piped up, "Can meditation help us see different faces of the divine, like Brahma and Brahman?"

Dad chuckled. "Perhaps. The divine can appear in many forms. Through meditation, you might feel calm and connected (combines calmness and connectedness), encountering Brahman. Or, you might find inspiration, a touch of Brahma, the creator."

The day unfolded with newfound purpose. Dad guided them through breathing exercises. It wasn't easy. Their minds wandered, filled with thoughts. But with encouragement and laughter, they persisted.

By the end, a peaceful stillness settled. They didn't see visions or have revelations, but there was a subtle shift — a sense of calm within, a quiet space in their minds.

"It wasn't a bright light," Saharsha said, "but a quiet feeling, like a gentle breeze."

Saumyaa agreed. "Peacefulness. Maybe the first glimpse of the divine light?"

Dad smiled. 'Perhaps, adventurers. Every journey starts with a step, and every path to Moksha begins with inner peace. The divine is always present, waiting to be discovered within. It's a journey, and you've just begun."

The seeds of curiosity were planted. Their quest to understand the divine had begun. Each meditation session, question, and story shared brought them closer to uncovering the universe's mysteries and their inner magic.

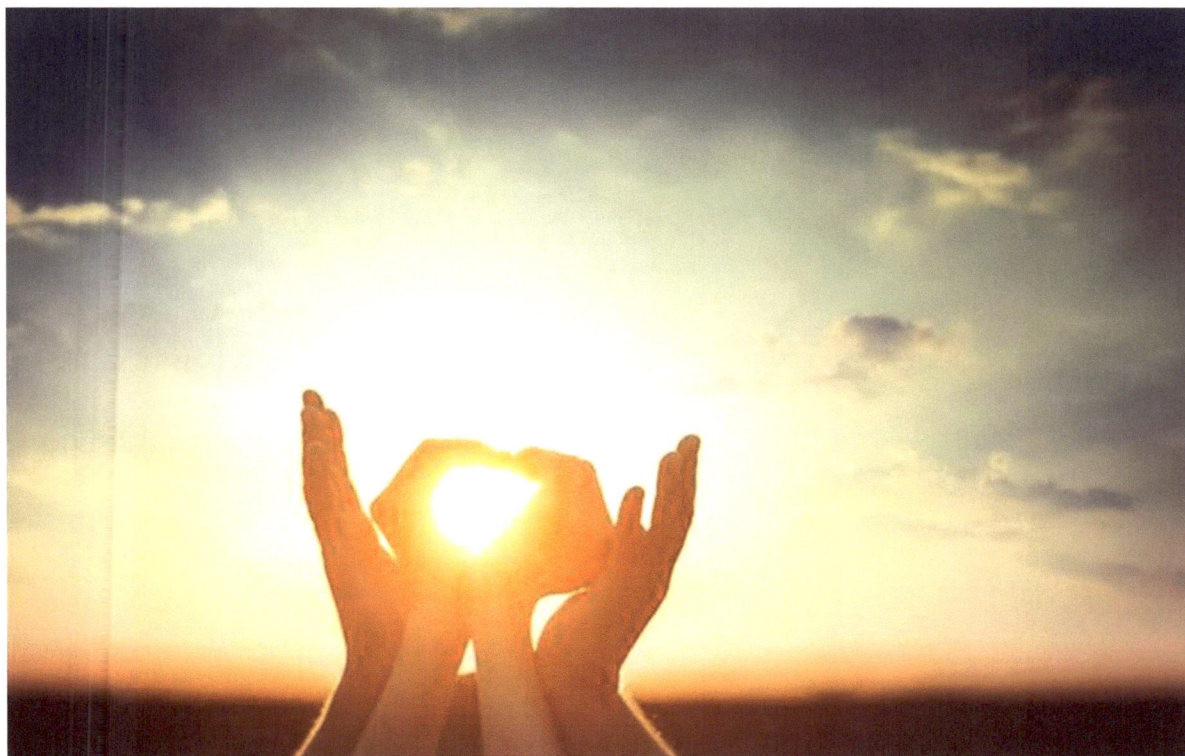

But the questions kept bubbling up.

"Dad," Saumyaa asked, "if everyone has this spark, why are some people mean? Is their spark dimmer?"

Saharsha chimed in, "And what about different religions? Do they worship the same light in different ways?"

Dad chuckled. "Great questions! Our exploration has just begun. Perhaps tomorrow, we can delve into good and evil, and how religions view the divine."

The next day, the afternoon sun lit the living room floor as Saumyaa and Saharsha awaited their discussion.

"Adventurers," Dad began, "ready to explore good and evil, and how religions perceive the divine?"

Saumyaa bounced. "Absolutely! Yesterday, you mentioned everyone having a divine spark. But if that's true, why are some people mean? Does it mean their spark is weaker?"

Dad stroked his chin. "That's a great question. The divine spark is pure, but a layer of dust, like negative thoughts or bad choices, can cloud it, leading to confusion and mean or selfish actions. It's like a flashlight – even the brightest one can be dimmed if the bulb is dirty."

Saharsha's eyes widened. "So, we have to keep our spark clean and bright?"

Dad nodded. "Exactly! Following your Dharma helps you live a good life and keeps your inner light shining."

"But what about different religions?" Saumyaa interjected. "At school, some kids talk about God, Allah, and many gods. Do they all worship the same divine light in different ways?"

Dad smiled. "Another fantastic question! Imagine the divine light as a vast ocean. Different religions approach it from various shores. Some see it as a personal God, while others view it as a universal force or many aspects of the divine. But ultimately, they all strive to connect with that same essence."

Saharsha scratched his head. "So, it's like looking at the same mountain from different sides?"

Dad chuckled. "A wonderful analogy! The important thing is to find what resonates with you, a path that helps you connect with the divine and live a meaningful life."

The conversation flowed with questions about religions and stories of compassion. Dad encouraged them to learn about other faiths, not to compare, but to appreciate the diverse ways humans seek the divine.

As the day ended, Saumyaa and Saharsha felt a new understanding. They realized the vastness of the universe was mirrored within them, with the potential for both darkness and light. But with meditation, self-awareness, and a growing understanding of the divine, they felt empowered to nurture their inner spark and illuminate their path.

"Dad," Saharsha asked before bed, "can we still have sleepovers with friends who have different beliefs?"

Dad smiled warmly. "Absolutely! Friendship and understanding are important parts of any path to the divine. Respecting others'

## CHAPTER SUMMARY: THE ETERNAL BRAHMA – A JOURNEY

Saumyaa and Saharsha's curiosity about the divine is ignited after a visit to the temple. Dad guides them through the concepts of Brahma, the creator, and Brahman, the universal spirit. They grapple with the idea of a single God versus many deities, and Dad explains how different religions might approach the same divine essence in various ways.

The chapter delves into the concept of Karma, the law of cause and effect, and how our choices shape our future. The discussion then explores the idea of **Moksha, liberation from the cycle of rebirth,** achieved through self-realization and connecting with the divine within.

The chapter concludes with a surge of questions in their minds. They ponder the nature of good and evil, the diverse beliefs of different religions, and the possibility of encountering the divine in a tangible way. Dad emphasizes the importance of the journey itself, the continuous exploration, and the power of small acts of kindness that honor the divine light within all beings.

Key themes explored:

- The nature of the divine in Hinduism (Brahma, Brahman)
- Karma and Moksha
- Meditation as a tool for self-discovery and inner peace
- Importance of questioning and exploring different beliefs
- Kindness and compassion as ways to connect with the divine

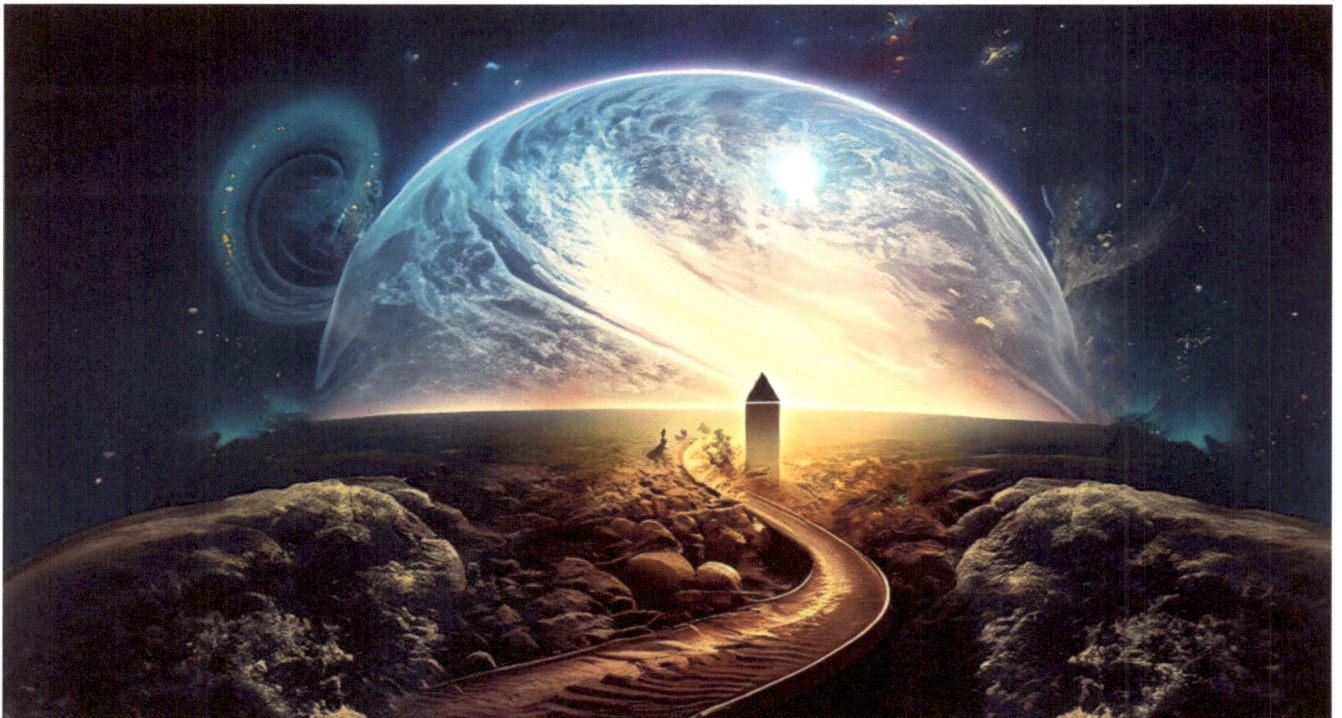

# Chapter 9: Discovering Divine Secrets
## The Journey to Supreme Knowledge

"

### *Awe-Inspiring Answers! Chapter 9: Divine Secrets*

*Eerie silence hangs in the air, replaced by the chirping of crickets. Saumyaa and Saharsha huddle closer, a million questions swirling in their curious minds.*

*What is God? Can we find Him everywhere? Join them on a remarkable quest for understanding!*

*Explore stories of Krishna's enchanting flute and Rama's unwavering strength. Learn how the divine can manifest in countless ways.*

*Is there a flicker of the divine within us all? Dad shares a heartwarming tale of a wise king and a tiny ant.*

Saumyaa and Saharsha practically bounced with excitement as Dad sat down for their usual evening chat about all things divine. The stories and ideas they'd explored lately had sparked a real curiosity in them, a burning desire to unravel the biggest mysteries of life.

"Dad," Saharsha blurted out, his eyes sparkling like stars, "if God can walk the earth, is He like us, or totally different?"

Dad chuckled, his smile crinkling at the corners. "That's a fantastic question, Saharsha! It's one that's been pondered by wise people for ages." He picked up a book from the shelf, its cover worn smooth and showing a picture of a bright sun. "Think of a block of clay," he started, flipping through the pages. "You can mold it into a cool animal, a funny mug, or even a whole plate. Each thing you make is different, but they're all still just clay in the end."

Saumyaa's brow furrowed in concentration. "So, you're saying God can take different shapes depending on where He appears?"

Dad nodded. "Exactly, Saumyaa. Some believe God is a single, unified reality, the source of all creation. Others believe He can manifest in various forms, like avatars, to guide humanity at different points in time."

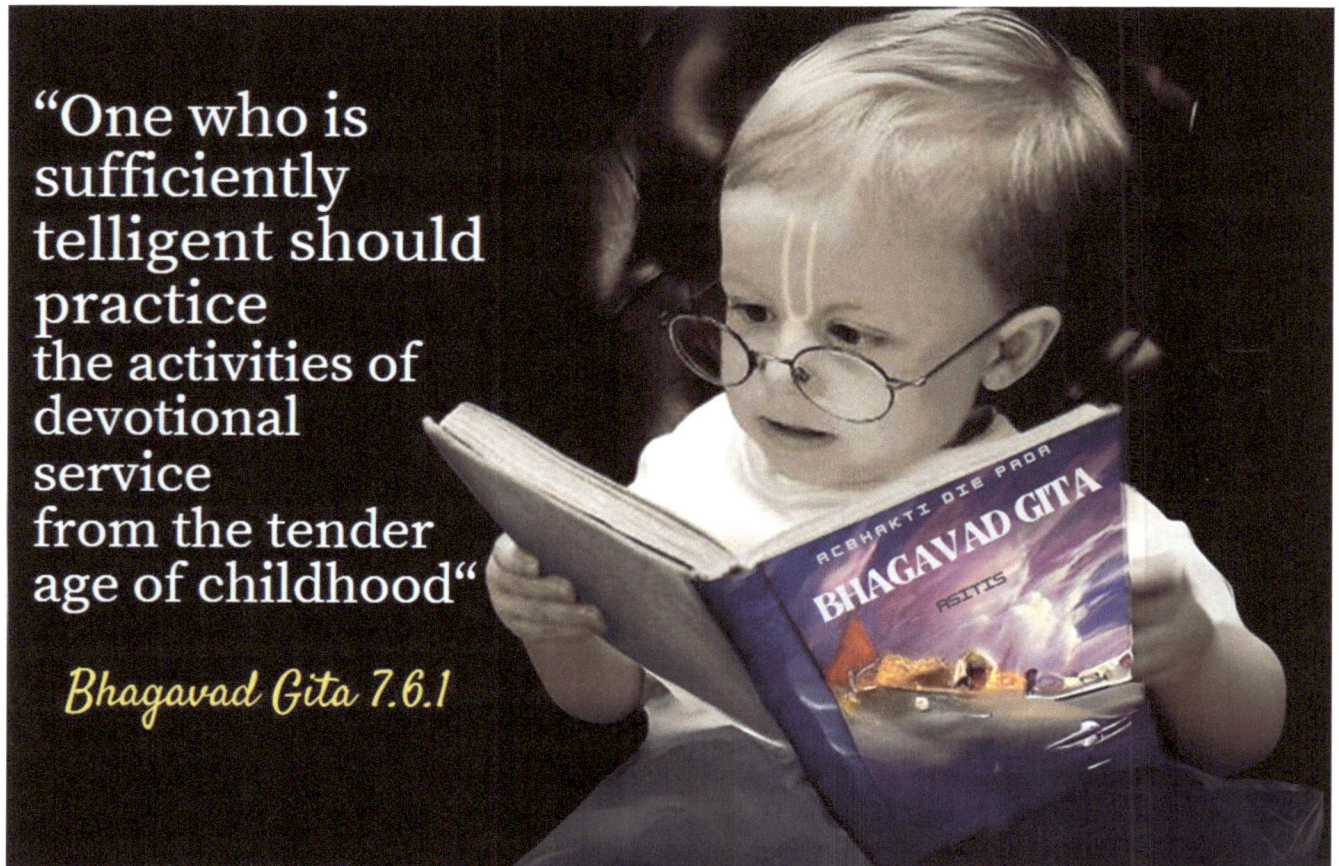

"One who is sufficiently telligent should practice the activities of devotional service from the tender age of childhood"

*Bhagavad Gita 7.6.1*

He delved into stories from the scriptures, tales filled with magic and wonder. They heard about Krishna, the fun-loving and strong god who played his flute, charming everyone who listened. They learned about Rama, the superhero of goodness, who faced tons of challenges without giving up, and his bow was like a symbol of his strength and fairness. Dad explained that according to Hindu religion, these avatars, or divine incarnations, like Krishna and Rama, descended to Earth to help humanity at different points in time, to restore dharma (righteousness) and defeat evil.

"But wait, Dad," Saharsha interrupted, his voice full of curiosity, "if God made everything, will everything turn back into God someday? Like melting all your gold jewelry into one big chunk again?"

Dad's eyes gleamed with appreciation. "A brilliant question, Saharsha! The universe is believed to undergo cycles of creation and destruction, a cosmic dance where everything dissolves back into the divine source, only to re-emerge in a new form."

Saumyaa's mind whirled with possibilities. "So, if God is everywhere and in everything," she pondered, her voice hushed with awe, "does that mean we can see Him in a tree or a flower?"

"Absolutely, Saumyaa!" Dad exclaimed. "Many traditions view the entire universe as a manifestation of the divine. When we appreciate the beauty of a sunrise or the strength of a mighty oak, we are connecting with that divine essence."

## THE WISE KING AND THE HUMBLE ANT

Dad smiled. "There's a beautiful story that perfectly demonstrates the concept of the divine spark within all living things," he began. "Once upon a time, there was a wise king, known for his fairness and kindness. He enjoyed taking walks in the palace gardens every day. One sunny afternoon, as he strolled past a flowerbed, he spotted a tiny ant struggling to carry a crumb that looked much bigger than itself."

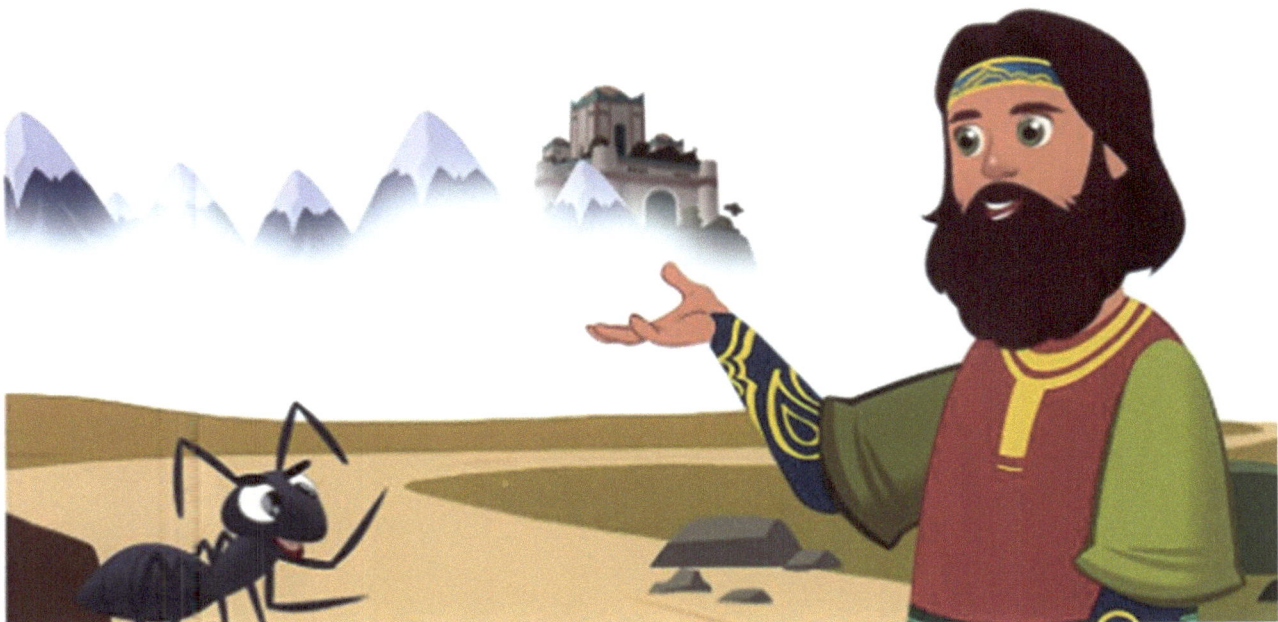

"The king, with a gentle heart, used his staff to nudge the crumb closer to an anthill, helping the little creature on its way."

"The ant, surprised by the unexpected help, looked up and saw the giant king standing above. It scurried up the king's leg and onto his hand. Then, in a surprising gesture, the ant carefully cleaned a tiny smudge on the king's royal ring. The king was touched. Even the smallest creature, he realized, could possess a divine spark, a light of kindness and helpfulness that shines within all of us."

Dad smiled warmly. "See, Saumyaa and Saharsha, the king's kindness and the ant's helpfulness are like tiny sparks of the divine light within each of them. It reminds us that no matter how big or small we are, we all have the potential for good."

Saumyaa's brow furrowed in thought. "So, the good things we do make our inner light shine brighter?"

Dad nodded. "Exactly! That's a wonderful way to think about it. In our lives, the choices we make are like seeds we plant. Good choices, like helping others or being kind, plant seeds that grow into positive experiences and happiness. This is the law of Karma, where our actions have consequences."

Saharsha tilted his head. "Karma sounds a bit scary. Does that mean if I made a mistake, I'll get punished?"

Dad chuckled. "Not exactly, Saharsha. Karma isn't about punishment, but about learning and growing. If you make a mistake, it's a chance to understand why it wasn't a good choice and do better next time. It's all part of the journey."

Saumyaa's eyes sparkled. "So, if we keep doing good things and making our inner light shine, can we break free from the cycle of being born again and again?"

Dad's eyes gleamed. "That's the idea behind Moksha, Saumyaa. By following your Dharma, living a good life, and nurturing your inner light, you can achieve liberation from the cycle of rebirth."

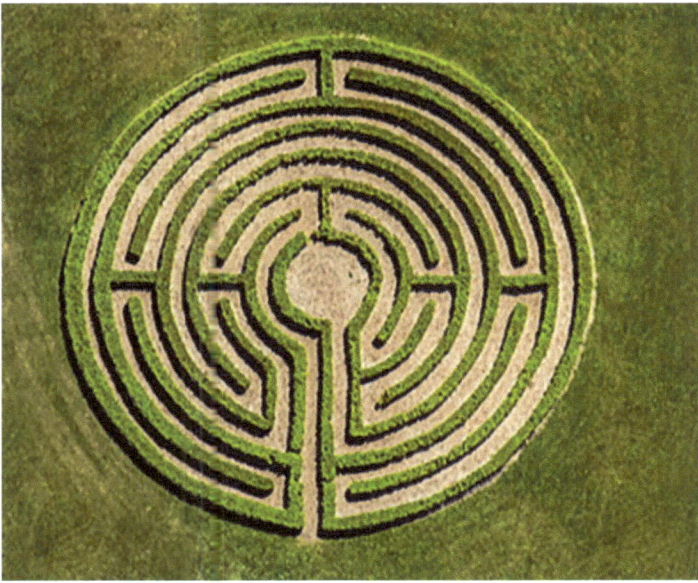

A comfortable silence settled upon them as Dad finished his story. Saharsha, his brow furrowed in thought, finally spoke. "But Dad, **if God is within us all, why doesn't everyone see it the same way? Why doesn't everyone love and worship Him?"**

Dad's gaze softened. "That's a wonderful question, Saharsha. Imagine a garden filled with different flowers. Each flower blooms in its own unique way, with its own color and fragrance. Yet, they all receive sunlight and nourishment from the same source. The divine light within us is like that sunlight. We all have it, but we experience and express it differently."

Saumyaa leaned forward, her eyes sparkling with a newfound determination. **"So, how can we cultivate that light within ourselves,** Dad? How can we feel it more?"

Dad smiled warmly. "There are many paths, Saumyaa. Meditation, prayer, and acts of kindness are all ways to connect with the divine spark within. Just like focusing sunlight through a magnifying glass can create warmth, focusing our attention inward can help us feel that inner light more clearly."

As they drifted off to sleep, their dreams were filled with celestial beings, shimmering lights, and a deep sense of awe. The vastness of the universe, once an intimidating mystery, now felt like a boundless playground of discovery. They knew their journey towards the divine had just begun, and with each question asked and each story shared, they felt themselves growing closer to the big mystery that enveloped them all.

The next morning, Saumyaa, ever the inquisitive one, bombarded Dad with more questions. "But Dad," she began, her brow furrowed in concentration, "what about all the different religions? Do they all worship the same God in different ways?"

## THE BLIND MEN AND THE ELEPHANT

To illustrate this point further, Dad began narrating a classic story: "There once lived a group of blind men in a village. One day, a magnificent elephant was brought to the village. Curious to let the blind men experience this wondrous creature, the villagers led each of them to touch a different part of the elephant."

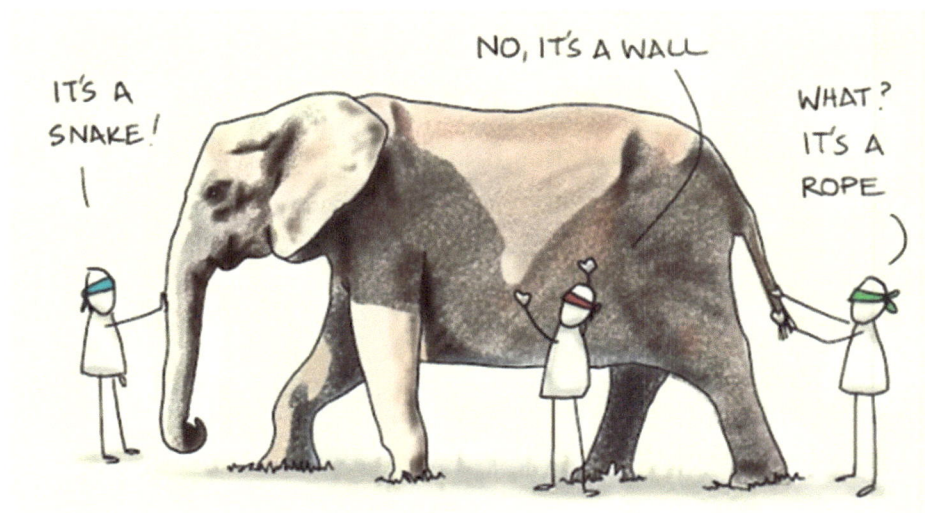

"The first blind man touched the elephant's trunk and declared, 'The elephant is like a thick snake!'"

"The second blind man, feeling the elephant's leg, exclaimed, 'No, it's a sturdy tree!'"

"The third man, grasping the elephant's side, insisted, 'It's a wall, smooth and flat!'"

Each blind man, based on their limited experience, had a different perception of the elephant. They argued amongst themselves, unable to understand the whole picture.

A wise man, observing their disagreement, approached them and explained, "You are all right, yet all wrong. Each of you has touched a part of the elephant, but none of you has experienced the whole creature."

Similarly, Dad explained, different religions might focus on different aspects of the divine. Some may emphasize God's power, others God's love, and still others God's wisdom. But just as the elephant is one magnificent being, the divine essence is ultimately one, even if experienced in diverse ways. This story highlights the importance of respecting different faiths and recognizing that they all may be seeking the same ultimate truth.

## THE LAMPLIGHT AND THE STARS

Dad continued, building upon the concept, "Imagine a group of travelers journeying through a vast desert at night. Feeling lost and disoriented, they stumble upon a hidden oasis. Relief washes over them as they see a welcoming lamplight flickering in the distance. '

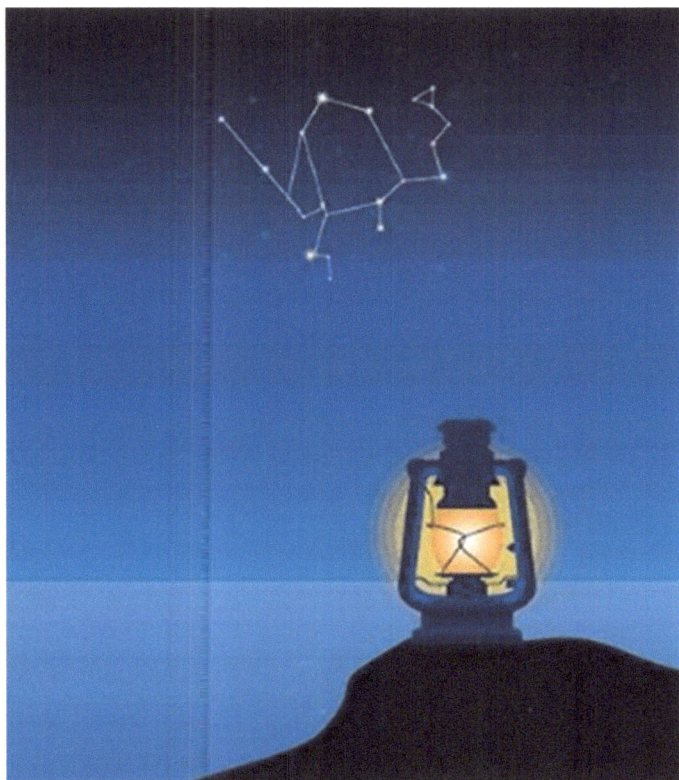

"Reaching the oasis, they discover a wellspring of cool water and a grove of fruit trees. They thank the kind hermit who resides there for his hospitality. The travelers then ask the hermit about the source of the lamplight. The hermit explains it's just a simple oil lamp, providing a beacon of comfort in the darkness."

"Later that night, one of the travelers gazes up at the breathtaking expanse of stars. In awe, they ask the hermit about the stars' significance. The hermit smiles and explains that the stars are a magnificent display of the universe's vastness and wonder."

"The next morning, the travelers prepare to depart. They thank the hermit once again, feeling grateful for his kindness and guidance. One traveler, curious, asks the hermit if the lamplight and the stars are connected."

The hermit chuckled. "They both illuminate the darkness in different ways, my friend. The lamp provides a warm, immediate comfort, while the stars offer a sense of awe and perspective. Both serve a purpose, just as different religions offer different paths to understand the divine light that shines within us all."

Dad concluded, "The important thing is to find a path that resonates with your heart, Saumyaa. As you explore different traditions, remember that the divine essence you seek may be the same light that guides and inspires others, even if it appears under a different name or form."

The depth of Dad's explanation sparked even more questions in Saharsha's mind. "But Dad," he said, his voice thoughtful, "if the divine spark is within us, can't bad things happen because of it too? Can darkness come from the same place as light?"

Dad smiled, acknowledging the complexity of Saharsha's question. "An excellent point, Saharsha. The divine spark within us grants us immense potential, the potential for great love, compassion, and creativity. But it also gives us the freedom to choose differently. Just like a fire can be used for warmth or destruction, the divine spark within us can manifest as positive or negative actions."

"So, how do we make sure we use it for good?" Saumyaa inquired, her voice filled with a newfound determination.

Dad's eyes twinkled with pride. **"That's the million-dollar question,** Saumyaa! It's a lifelong journey of learning and self-discovery. Here are a few ways to nurture the good within your divine spark:"

- **Practice kindness:** Look for opportunities to help others, big or small. A kind word, a helping hand, or simply listening with a compassionate heart can make a difference. Remember, even the smallest acts of kindness can ripple outwards, creating a wave of positivity.

- **Cultivate gratitude:** Take time each day to appreciate the good things in your life, no matter how ordinary they may seem. Gratitude reminds you of the blessings you have and keeps your heart open to the beauty around you.

- **Follow your conscience:** That inner voice, that gut feeling, is often your divine spark guiding you. When faced with a difficult choice, pause and listen to what feels right. It may not always be the easiest path, but it will lead you closer to the light within.

- **Explore different practices:** Meditation, prayer, spending time in nature – there are many ways to connect with your inner self. Experiment and find what resonates with you. As you connect with your inner light, it will naturally illuminate the path ahead.

"Remember," Dad continued, his voice warm, "you are not alone on this journey. There are countless stories, traditions, and wise teachings that can offer guidance. Learn from them, question them, and ultimately, discover your own unique path to nurturing the divine spark within you."

The night deepened, filled with the quiet hum of crickets and the soft glow of the moon peeking through their window. Saumyaa and Saharsha, their minds brimming with newfound knowledge and a sense of purpose, snuggled deeper into their beds. They knew their exploration of the divine had just begun, but with each step, they felt a growing sense of connection to the vast mystery that surrounded them. They dreamt of shimmering lights, helping hands, and a warmth that emanated from deep within, a constant reminder of the divine spark that resided within them, waiting to be nurtured and shared with the world.

## CHAPTER SUMMARY: THE JOURNEY TO SUPREME KNOWLEDGE

Saumyaa and Saharsha's curiosity about the divine deepens as they explore the concept with their Dad. Through captivating stories and thought-provoking questions, they delve into themes like:

- **The Divine in Different Forms:** Dad uses the metaphor of gold being shaped into different objects to explain how the divine essence can manifest in various ways, like avatars in different religions. Stories of Krishna and Rama illustrate this concept.

- **The Cycle of Creation and Destruction:** The universe is believed to undergo cycles where everything dissolves back into the divine source and re-emerges in a new form. This is likened to melting gold jewelry back into a single piece.

- **The Divine Spark Within:** Everything in the universe is a manifestation of the divine. Experiencing beauty in nature or appreciating the world around us is a way to connect with this divine spark.

Dad uses stories to illustrate further:

- **The Wise King and the Humble Ant:** Even the smallest creatures can demonstrate the divine spark through their actions.

Respecting Different Religions:

- **The Blind Men and the Elephant:** Each blind man's limited experience with the elephant represents how different religions focus on various aspects of the same divine essence.

- **The Lamplight and the Stars:** Both the lamp and the stars offer different yet valuable ways to illuminate the darkness, just like different religions offer diverse paths to understanding the divine within.

## Finding Your Path:

- Dad emphasizes the importance of finding a spiritual path that resonates with each individual. Exploring different traditions and practices can help with this discovery.

## Nurturing the Divine Spark:

- Dad offers practical ways to nurture the good within the divine spark, such as practicing kindness, cultivating gratitude, following your conscience, and exploring different spiritual practices.

## Chapter Ends with a Sense of Wonder:

Saumyaa and Saharsha feel a growing connection to the divine mystery and a sense of purpose in nurturing their own divine spark. They dream of a future filled with light, kindness, and a deeper understanding of their place in the universe.

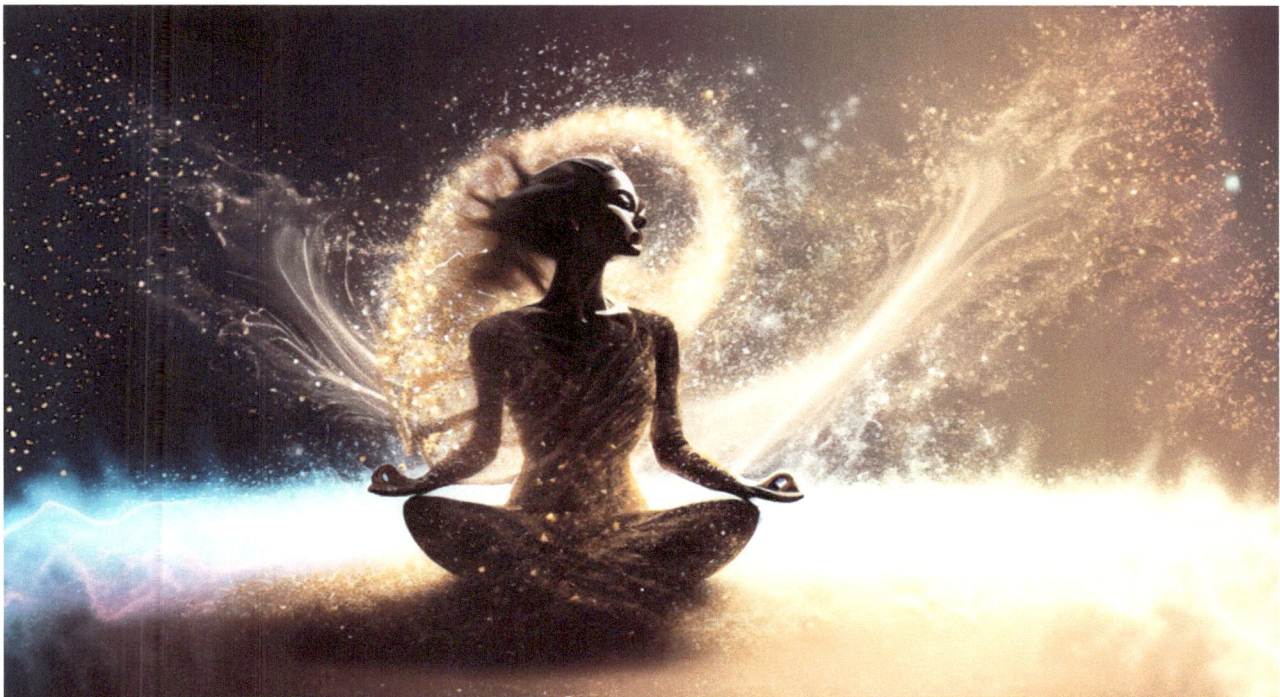

# Chapter 10: God's Many Forms

## Exploring Divine Manifestations

"

### Awe-Inspiring Answers! God's Many Forms

*Warm fireflies dance in the twilight, casting an otherworldly glow on Saumyaa and Saharsha's faces. Their eyes sparkle with a thousand questions.*
*Can one God appear in countless forms? Join them on a captivating quest to discover the divine in all its glory!*
*Explore tales of Vishnu, the protector, and Shiva, the mighty force of creation and destruction. Learn how the divine can take shape in countless ways, like a single ray of light splitting into a dazzling spectrum.*
*Is there a spark of the divine within us all? Dad ignites their curiosity with a story unlike any other.*
*Chapter 10: Embrace the Divine in All Its Forms! Explore God's Many Faces!*

The flickering flames of the diyas (oil lamp made from clay) cast a warm glow on the faces of Saumyaa and Saharsha as they huddled around Dad on the rug. The previous stories about Krishna and Rama lingered in their minds, sparking a fire of curiosity.

"Dad," blurted out Saharsha, his voice filled with wonder, "**if God can come to Earth, is He the same as us, or completely different?**"

Dad chuckled, his warm smile crinkling the corners of his eyes. "That's a fantastic question, Saharsha. It's a question that has puzzled philosophers and wise p for centuries." He reached for a book on the shelf, its worn cover adorned with an image of a radiant sun. "Imagine a piece of gold," he began, flipping through the pages. "It can be fashioned into a necklace, a ring, or a shimmering coin. Each form is different, yet they are all ultimately gold."

Saumyaa's brow furrowed in concentration. "So, you're saying God can take different shapes depending on where He appears?"

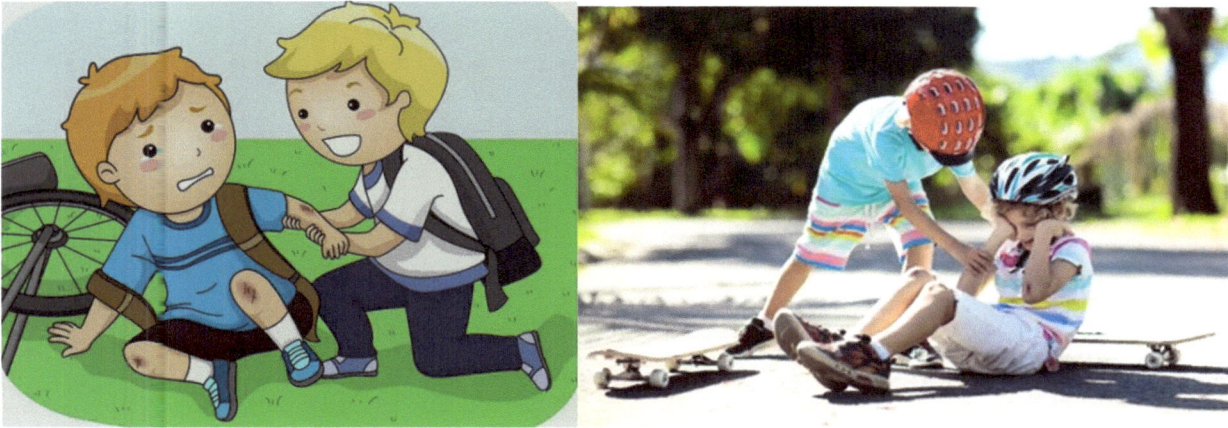

Dad nodded. "Exactly, Saumyaa. There are different beliefs about how God interacts with the world. Some people imagine God as a single, all-powerful universal source, kind of like the first spark that started everything. Others believe God can take different shapes, like superheroes appearing to help people in times of need. These special forms are called avatars."

He then launched into exciting stories from their scriptures, filled with adventure and wonder. They learned about Vishnu, the protector, who, like a mighty guardian, keeps the world safe from harm through his different avatars. They also heard about Shiva, the powerful force who can both create and destroy, kind of like a giant artist who keeps remaking the world even more beautiful!

"But Dad," Saharsha chimed in, his voice brimming with curiosity, "if everything comes from God, then will everything eventually become God again? Like melting gold jewelry back into a single piece?"

Dad's eyes gleamed with appreciation. "A brilliant question, Saharsha! The universe is believed to undergo cycles of creation and destruction, a cosmic dance where everything dissolves back into the divine source, only to re-emerge in a new form."

Saumyaa's mind whirled with possibilities. "So, if God is everywhere and in everything," she pondered, her voice hushed with awe, "does that mean we can see Him in a tree or a flower?"

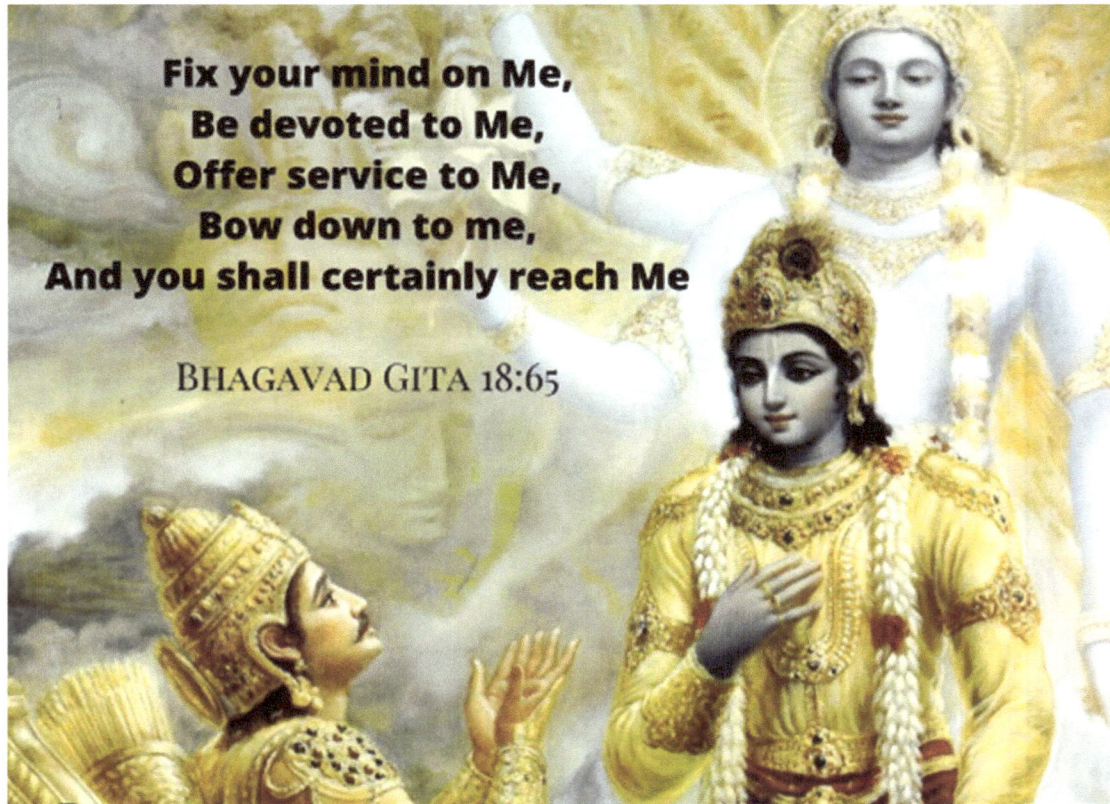

Fix your mind on Me,
Be devoted to Me,
Offer service to Me,
Bow down to me,
And you shall certainly reach Me

BHAGAVAD GITA 18:65

"Absolutely, Saumyaa!" Dad exclaimed. "Many traditions view the entire universe as a manifestation of the Divine. When we appreciate the beauty of a sunrise or the strength of a mighty oak, we are connecting with that divine essence."

## THE PAINTER AND THE MOUNTAIN

Dad chuckled. "There's a beautiful story that perfectly captures the idea of God existing in different forms," he began. "Once upon a time, there was a famous painter, known for his stunning pictures of nature. He traveled to a peaceful village nestled beneath a towering mountain."

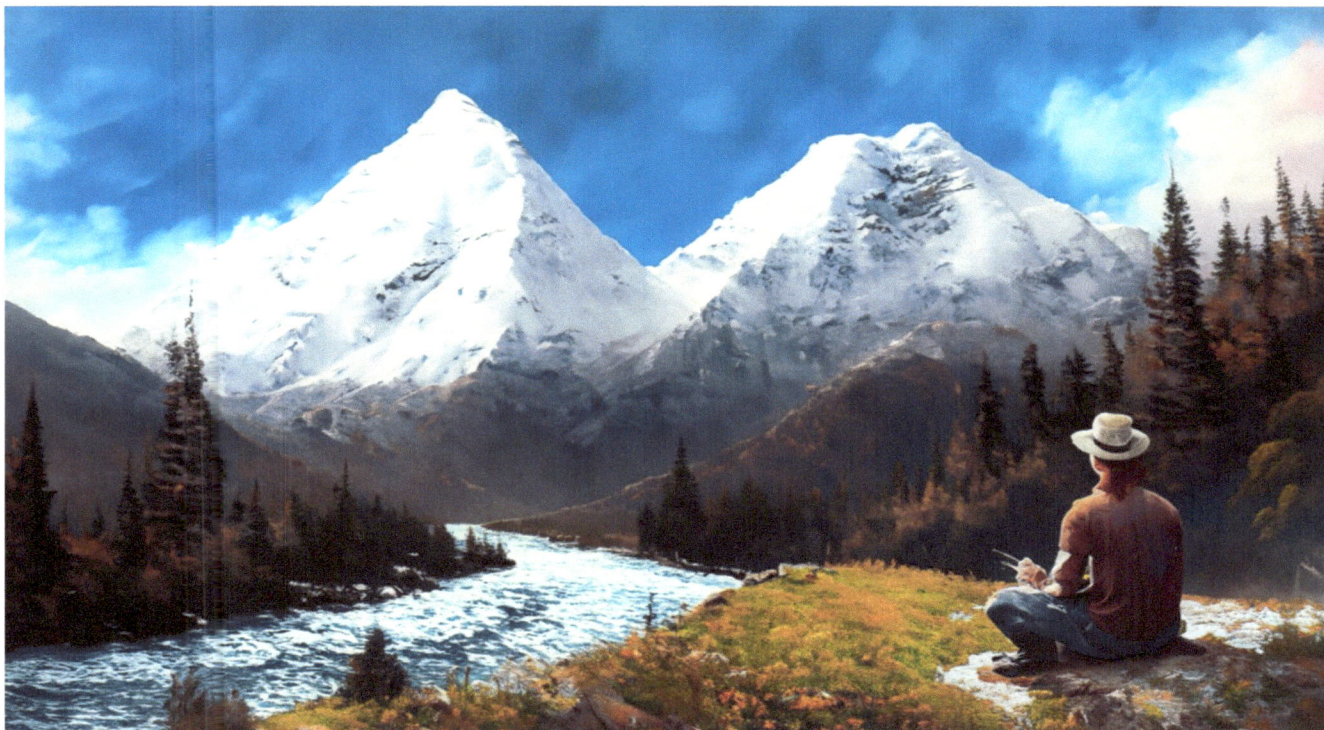

"The next morning, eager to capture the mountain's majesty, he set out with his paints and brushes. He found a perfect spot and began to paint, his brushstrokes bringing the mountain to life on his canvas.

As he focused on the details, a curious child from the village approached him and asked, 'Mister, are you painting the fluffy white clouds, the green trees, or the big grey rocks?'"

The painter smiled warmly. "That's a great question! I'm painting the whole mountain, my friend. The clouds, the trees, and the rocks are all part of what makes the mountain so special. By capturing them all, I hope to show the true beauty of the mountain itself.'"

"Similarly," Dad explained, "when we experience the wonders of the universe, we are connecting with the divine essence that permeates all of creation."

A comfortable silence settled upon them as Dad finished his captivating story. Saharsha, his brow furrowed in thought, finally spoke. "But Dad, if God is within us all, why doesn't everyone see it the same way? Why doesn't everyone love and worship Him?"

Dad's gaze softened. "That's a wonderful question, Saharsha. Remember the story of the painter and the mountain? Just like the child saw different parts of the mountain, people might focus on different aspects of the divine light within us."

Dad smiled warmly. "Exactly, Saumyaa! Some people might connect with God through the beauty of nature, like the artist appreciating the mountain's awesomeness. Others might feel a deep connection by helping others, like a superhero spreading kindness!"

Saharsha tilted his head. "So, there are many ways to see the special light inside us?"

Dad nodded. "There are many paths, Saharsha. Some people find God through prayer and talking to Him, while others experience the divine through music or creating something beautiful. The important thing is to find what makes you feel good and happy inside, a way to connect with that special spark."

Saumyaa leaned forward, her eyes sparkling with a newfound determination. "So, how do we make that light inside us shine brighter, Dad? How do we feel it more?"

Dad smiled warmly. "There are many ways, Saumyaa. Taking quiet moments to calm your mind, like sitting still and focusing on your breath, acts of kindness, and simply appreciating the cool breeze or a funny animal can all help us connect with the divine spark within. Remember, the journey itself is a kind of adventure, a constant exploration of the biggest mystery of all!"

Thinking ahead:

Dad's smile crinkled at the corners again. "Tomorrow, we can explore some of these adventures in more detail. Perhaps we can even try a short meditation together, like becoming a superhero of stillness for a few minutes! Who knows, maybe we'll even discover some of your own special ways to make your inner light shine!"

Saumyaa, ever the inquisitive one, pressed further. "But Dad," she began, her brow furrowed in thought, "if the divine spark is within us, can't bad things happen because of it too? Can darkness come from the same place as light?"

Dad's eyes gleamed with pride at his daughter's thoughtful question. "An excellent point, Saumyaa. The divine spark within us grants us amazing power, the power for great love, kindness, and creativity. But it also gives us the freedom to choose differently. Just like a fire can be used to keep us warm or to burn things down, the divine spark within us can show itself in good or bad ways."

Saharsha, the more analytical of the two, chimed in with a question that had been bubbling in his mind. "So, if we have this divine spark, why do we have to learn about it or practice anything? Shouldn't that connection just be there naturally?"

Dad chuckled "A great question, Saharsha! The divine spark is always there, like a tiny flicker in our hearts. But like any flicker, it needs care to grow into a bright flame. Through things like prayer, meditation, and doing good deeds, we help that tiny flicker grow bigger, letting its light shine on us and everyone around us."

Saumyaa pondered this for a moment, then asked another question that surprised Dad with its depth. "But Dad, if everyone has this divine spark, wouldn't that mean everyone is naturally kind?"

Dad's smile softened. "That's a beautiful thought, Saumyaa. Perhaps everyone is born with the ability to be kind. But as we grow up, the world around us can influence us, with all sorts of experiences and choices. Sometimes, those influences can make it hard to see the good spark inside us clearly."

Saharsha, ever the pragmatist, added his own perspective. "So, learning about the Divine and doing all these things is like wiping the dust off that spark and letting it shine again?"

Dad nodded, his heart swelling with pride at his children's insightful questions. "Exactly, Saharsha! It's about remembering the good that's already inside us and learning to show it in how we think, talk, and act. It's a lifelong adventure of learning about ourselves, and every step we take brings us closer to the light that shines within."

As the night deepened, the only sound was the gentle hum of the crickets and the soft glow of the diyas flickering on the floor. Saumyaa and Saharsha, their minds filled with wonder and a sense of purpose, snuggled deeper into their pillows. They knew their exploration of the Divine had just begun, but they were no longer afraid of the darkness. They carried within them the knowledge of the divine spark, a tiny ember waiting to be nurtured and shared with the world.

## CHAPTER SUMMARY: EXPLORING DIVINE MANIFESTATIONS

Saumyaa and Saharsha delve deeper into the concept of the Divine with their Dad. Through stories and discussions, they explore themes like:

- **Manifestations of the Divine:** The Divine can take various forms, like avatars, and is believed to be present throughout creation – in the beauty of nature, the strength of mountains, and even within ourselves.

- **The Divine Spark:** Dad uses the metaphor of a piece of gold being shaped into different forms to explain how the Divine can manifest in diverse ways.

Dad shares stories to illustrate:

- **The Painter and the Mountain:** This story highlights how appreciating the various aspects of creation – sky, trees, rocks – allows us to connect with the essence of the Divine that permeates it all.

Thoughtful Questions from the Children:

- **Saumyaa:** If the divine spark is within us, can darkness also come from it?

- **Saharsha:** If we have this divine spark, why do we need to learn about it? Shouldn't the connection be natural?

- **Saumyaa:** If everyone has this divine spark, wouldn't everyone be inherently good?

- **Saharsha:** Learning about the Divine and practicing spiritual activities is like cleaning the dust off that spark and letting it shine again?

Key Takeaways:

- The Divine spark within us grants us immense potential for good and creativity, but also the freedom to choose differently.

- Practices like prayer, meditation, and good deeds help nurture the divine spark within us, allowing it to illuminate our lives and the world around us.

- Everyone has the potential for good, but external influences can cloud the divine spark. Learning about the Divine and practicing spiritual activities helps us reconnect with that inherent goodness.

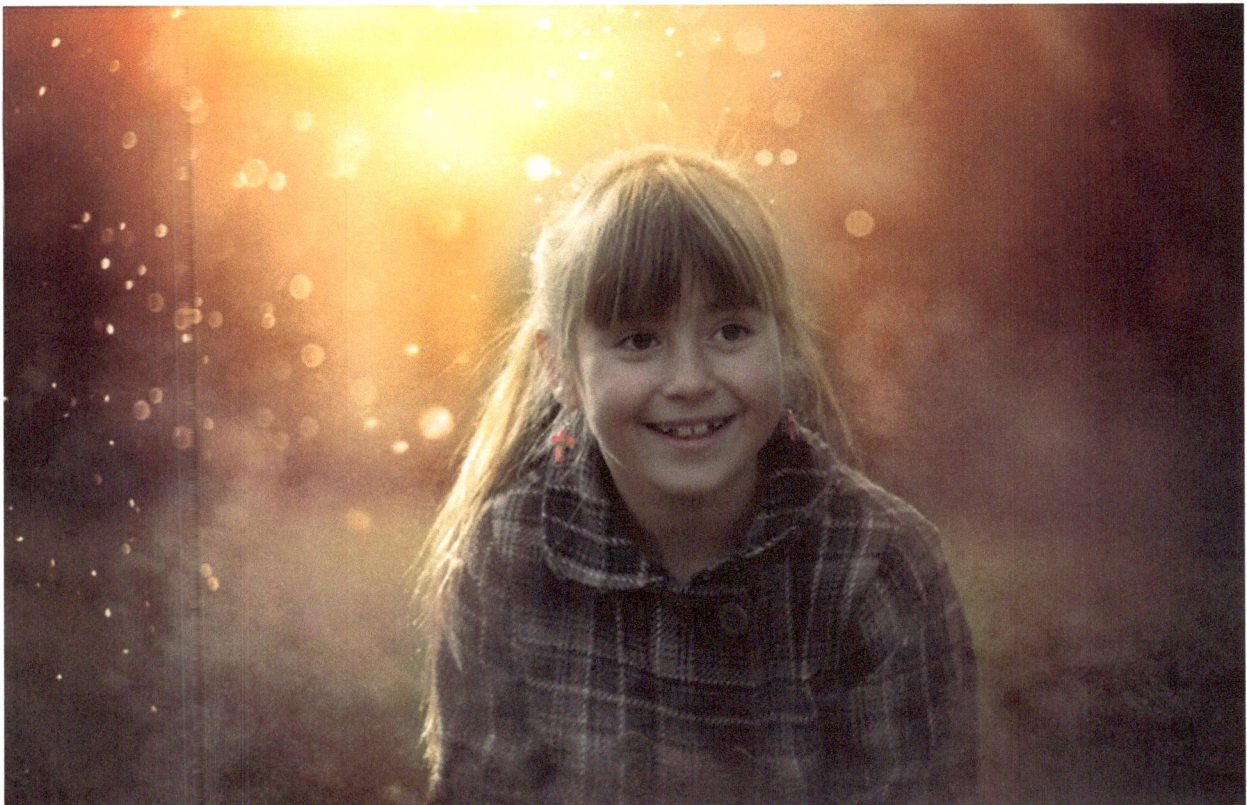

*A child looking at a beautiful sunset, recognizing the divine in nature's beauty.*

# Chapter 11: Divine Sight
## Beholding the Vision of God

*Divine Sight – Beholding the Vision of God*

*Can we truly see the Divine? Join them on a captivating quest to unveil the mysteries of inner vision!*
*Explore traditions that speak of visions and dreams, encounters that spark a deeper connection with the Divine essence. Learn how practices like meditation can act as a key, unlocking a doorway to a world unseen.*
*Is there a way to perceive the Divine spark more clearly? Dad ignites their curiosity with a story that will illuminate the night.*

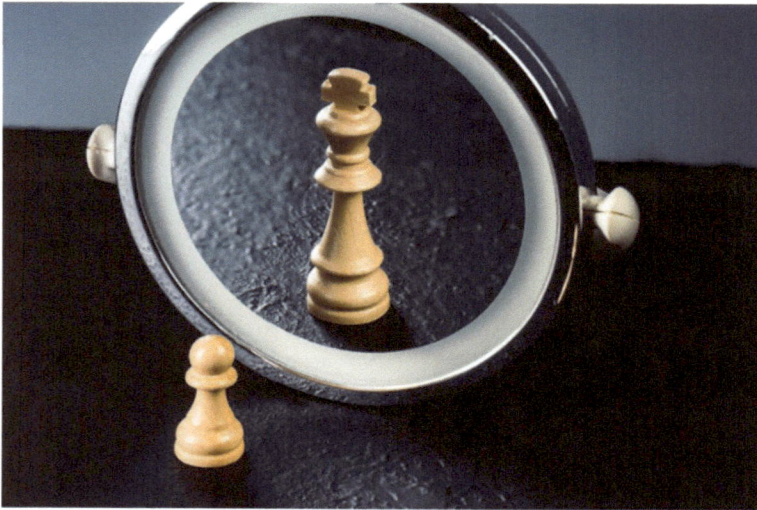

The embers in the fireplace crackled softly, casting dancing shadows on the walls as Saharsha and Saumyaa snuggled closer to Dad. Their young minds were abuzz with questions after learning about the Divine spark within all creation.

"Dad," Saumyaa began, her voice filled with a child's innocent curiosity, "you said the Divine can appear in visions. Can we actually see God?"

Dad's eyes softened with understanding. "That's a wonderful question, Saumyaa. Many traditions believe God isn't limited to a physical form we can see with our eyes."

He reached for a book on the shelf, its pages whispering tales of ancient wisdom. "Imagine the vast ocean," Dad said, opening the book. "We can't see the entire ocean at once, but we can experience its presence through the waves lapping at the shore or a single glistening drop of water. In the same way, the Divine presence permeates the universe, but we might not always perceive it directly."

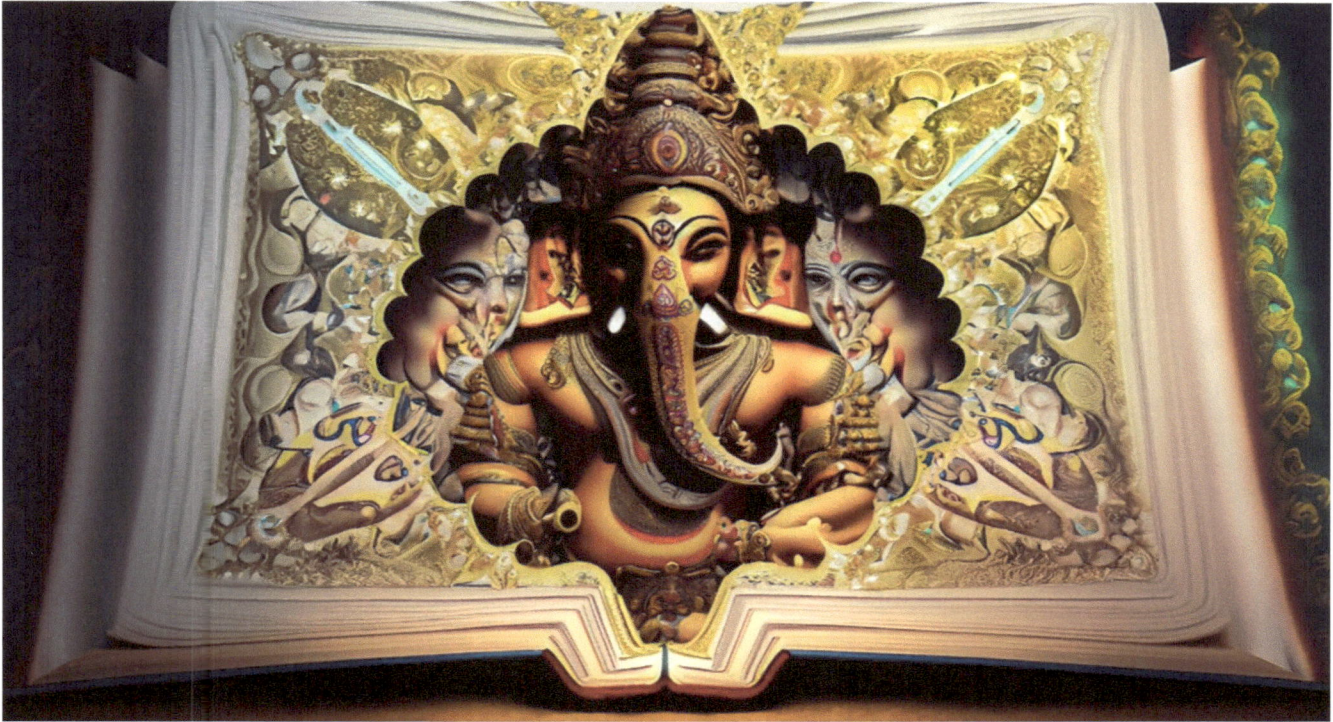

Saharsha's brow furrowed in concentration. "So, we can't see God directly, but we can sense Him in everything around us? Like, if we pay attention really closely, can we feel the Divine spark in a flower or a ladybug?"

Dad smiled warmly. "Exactly, Saharsha! Some believe the Divine presence permeates the universe, like the ocean's essence flowing through every drop. When we appreciate the beauty of a sunrise or the intricate details of a flower, we are connecting with that very essence. It's like opening our hearts and minds to a deeper reality that exists beyond the physical world."

## THE ALCHEMIST AND THE GOLDEN SEED

To explain what an alchemist was, Dad began a captivating story. "Imagine a scientist, but way back in old times, someone who loved figuring things out and believed in the magic hidden in the world. These special scientists were called alchemists. They spent their days in workshops experimenting with all sorts of things, trying to turn ordinary objects into something extraordinary – like gold!"

Dad chuckled. "They weren't always successful, but their curiosity and experiments helped pave the way for the science we know today. Now, listen to the tale of a very special alchemist..."

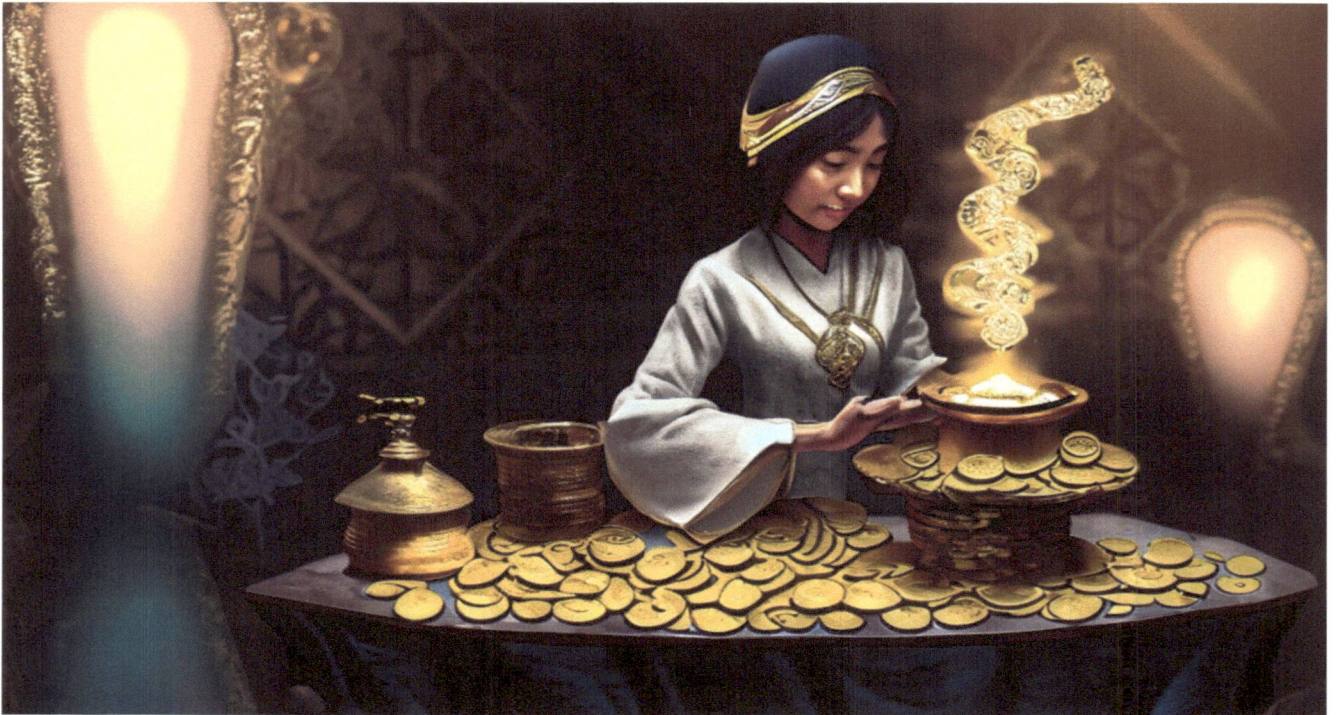

A young alchemist named Maya was known for her curiosity and her yearning to understand the secrets of the universe. One day, on a journey through a mystical forest, she stumbled upon a hidden grove bathed in an otherworldly glow. In the center stood a magnificent tree, unlike any she had ever seen, its leaves shimmering with an ethereal light.

Intrigued, Maya approached the tree and noticed a single, golden seed nestled amongst its leaves. As she picked it up, a sense of awe washed over her. She felt a connection to something far greater than herself, a sense of the Divine spark that pulsed within the universe and within the golden seed itself.

"This seed," Maya whispered, her voice filled with reverence, "holds within it the potential for something extraordinary."

Maya carefully planted the seed in her garden, nurturing it with love and care. As days turned into weeks, a sprout emerged from the soil, unlike any plant she had ever seen. Its leaves shimmered with a faint, golden light, a constant reminder of the extraordinary potential that lay within.

One evening, as Dad finished tucking them in, Saumyaa, her eyes sparkling with curiosity, asked, "But Dad, what happened to the golden seed? Did it grow into a magical tree?"

Dad smiled warmly. "That's a wonderful question, Saumyaa. The story tells us that the seed held the potential for something extraordinary. But what that extraordinary thing was, is left to our imagination."

Saharsha, the more analytical one, chimed in, "So, the story is about possibility, not a specific outcome?"

Dad nodded. "Exactly, Saharsha. Just like the golden seed, each of us has the potential for something extraordinary within us. It could be a talent for music, a passion for helping others, or simply the ability to spread kindness. The important thing is to nurture that potential, like Maya nurturing the seed, so our inner light can shine brightly."

Saumyaa pondered this for a moment, then a thoughtful expression crossed her face. "So, the divine spark is like that golden seed, Dad? It has the potential to grow into something amazing?"

Dad's heart swelled with pride. "A beautiful thought, Saumyaa! The divine spark is like that seed, holding the potential for love, compassion, and creativity. By practicing kindness, following our dreams, and connecting with the world around us, we can help that spark grow and make the world a more beautiful place."

As they drifted off to sleep, Saumyaa and Saharsha dreamt of golden seeds sprouting within them, radiating a warm, golden light. They knew their journey of nurturing their inner spark had just begun, and they were filled with a sense of excitement and possibility.

## GENERAL AND THOUGHT-PROVOKING QUESTIONS:

### 1. Saumyaa's Curiosity:

Saumyaa's brow furrowed in thought. "Dad, the Divine is everywhere, right? So, isn't it strange that some people have special experiences like visions or dreams where they feel closer to God? Maybe these experiences happen when our hearts and minds are more open to feeling the Divine essence?"

Dad's eyes gleamed with pride at his daughter's insightful question. "Excellent point, Saumyaa! You're absolutely right. Some believe that practices like meditation, prayer, and acts of kindness can purify our hearts and minds, making us more receptive to the Divine presence on a deeper level. Perhaps visions and dreams are glimpses of this deeper connection, a way of experiencing the Divine spark ignite within us."

### 2. Saharsha's Inquiry:

"Do animals feel the Divine presence too, Dad? Even though they can't talk or pray?" Saharsha tilted his head, pondering the concept.

Dad chuckled. "An interesting thought, Saharsha. Some traditions believe the Divine spark exists in all living things, not just humans. Perhaps animals experience the Divine in their own way, through their connection to nature and their instincts."

## The Conversation Deepens:

The conversation continued late into the night, exploring themes of devotion and its role in connecting with the Divine. Dad explained how selfless service could purify the heart, making it more receptive to experiencing the Divine presence.

## A Moment of Reflection:

As Dad finished a captivating story, a comfortable silence settled. Saumyaa, her eyes sparkling with newfound understanding, spoke first. "So, Dad, even though we can't see God with our eyes, we can feel His presence everywhere if we open our hearts?"

Dad's face lit up with pride. "Absolutely, Saumyaa! By cultivating devotion, practicing good deeds, and appreciating the wonders of the world, we can cultivate a sense of awe and reverence. This allows us to connect with the Divine presence that flows through all things."

## Saharsha's Question and a Deeper Explanation:

Saharsha, ever the pragmatist, chimed in with a thoughtful question. "But Dad, if the Divine is everywhere, why do some people say they've seen Him in visions or dreams?"

Dad chuckled gently. "That's a question many have pondered, Saharsha. Some believe that intense devotion and meditation can purify the mind, allowing for glimpses of the Divine in a non-physical way. These visions might not be literal sightings of God, but rather a heightened awareness of the Divine essence that permeates everything."

## Saumyaa's Insight:

Saumyaa's eyes widened with wonder. "So, maybe the visions aren't about seeing God with our eyes, but about feeling His presence more deeply? Like a flower blooming and releasing its fragrance, the visions might be a way for the Divine spark within us to express itself more fully?"

Dad beamed. "A brilliant thought, Saumyaa! Perhaps visions are a way of experiencing the Divine that transcends the limitations of our physical senses. They might be a confirmation of our connection to something far greater than ourselves."

## Thought-provoking Prompt:

Dad looked at his children, their faces glowing in the warm firelight.

"Now, here's a question for both of you to ponder. If the Divine spark exists within all living things, and experiencing the Divine is about opening our hearts and minds, how can we approach the world in a way that honors and connects with the Divine spark in everything around us?"

Saharsha and Saumyaa fell silent, their young minds brimming with newfound questions and a burgeoning sense of wonder. They knew their exploration of the Divine mystery was far from over, but tonight, they carried with them the knowledge that the Divine presence wasn't something distant and unapproachable. It was a spark within them, a vibrant essence woven into the very fabric of their world, waiting to be nurtured and explored.

## CHAPTER SUMMARY: DIVING SIGHT

Saumyaa and Saharsha delve deeper into the concept of experiencing the Divine with their Dad. Through stories and discussions, they explore themes like:

- **Indirect Experience of the Divine:** The Divine isn't limited to a physical form and can't be directly seen with our eyes.

- **Divine Presence in Everything:** The Divine essence permeates the universe, like the ocean flows through every drop. We can connect with it by appreciating the beauty of nature or the intricate details of creation.

- **Visions and Dreams:** Some people report experiencing the Divine in visions or dreams. These might not be literal sightings, but a heightened awareness of the Divine spark within and around us.

- The story of the alchemist, Maya, finding a golden seed in a mystical grove, symbolizes discovering the Divine spark within the universe and ourselves.

## General & Thought-Provoking Questions:

- **Saumyaa:** If the Divine is everywhere, why do some have special experiences like visions or dreams?

- **Saharsha:** Can animals feel the Divine presence too?

## Dad's Answers:

- Visions and dreams could be a way of experiencing the Divine more deeply when our hearts and minds are open.

- The Divine spark might exist in all living things, and animals experience it in their own way.

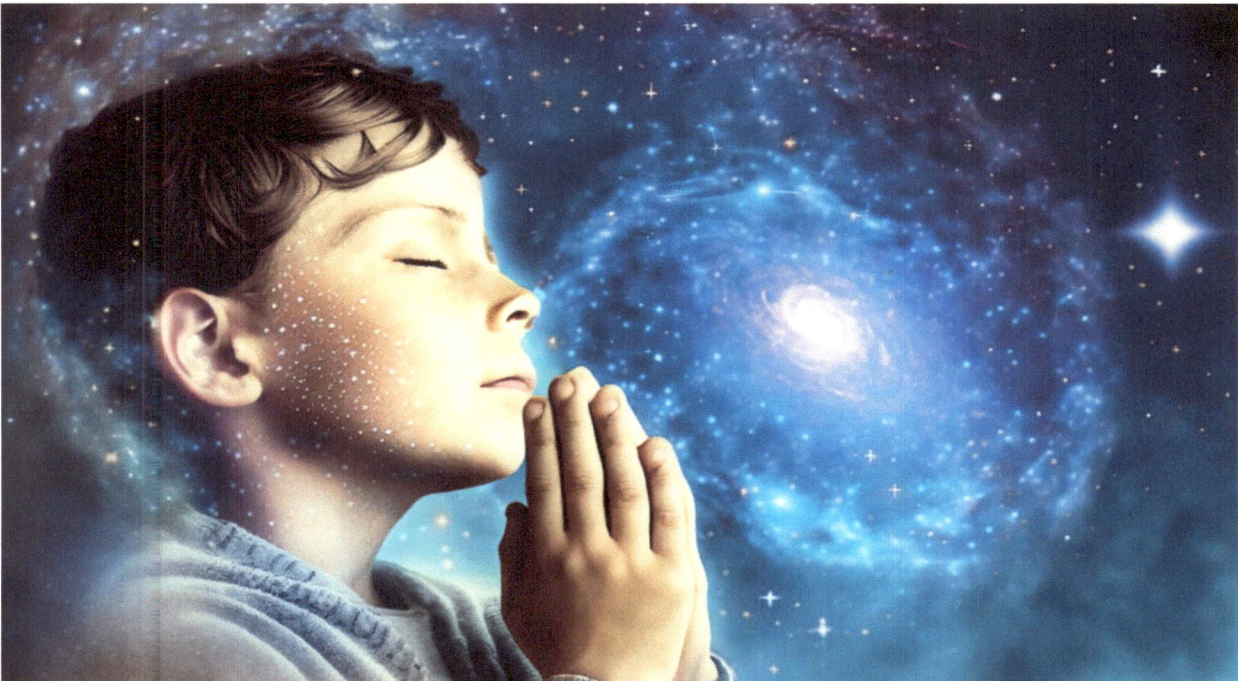

*A child with closed eyes representing inner vision and intuition.*

# Chapter 12: The Path of Devotion (Bhakti)

**"**

*Can we truly feel the Divine presence within us?*

*Join the family on a heartfelt exploration to discover the whispers of the Divine in their own hearts!*
*Delve into ancient wisdom that speaks of devotion's power to awaken the Divine spark. Explore stories of saints and seekers who cultivated a deep inner connection through love and bhakti.*
*Is there a way to nurture the Divine flame within? Dad kindles their curiosity with a tale that will illuminate their journey inward.*
*Chapter 12: The Path of Devotion (Bhakti) – Unveil the Divine Within!*

The cozy living room was bathed in the warm glow of the fireplace as Saharsha and Saumyaa snuggled closer to Dad. Their young minds buzzed with questions after learning about the power of prayer and meditation.

"Dad," Saumyaa began, her voice filled with curiosity, "Grandma said we should pray or meditate every day. Is that like a chore, or a way to connect with the Divine?"

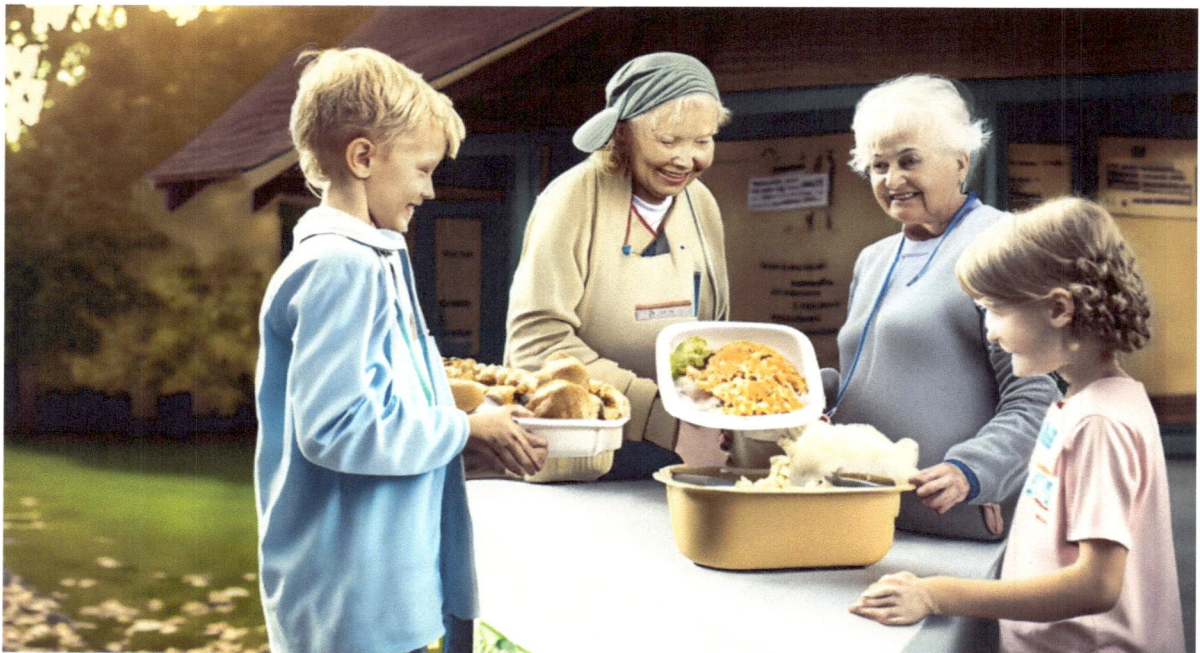

Dad smiled warmly. "It's a wonderful question, Saumyaa. Think of it less like a chore and more like spending time with a loved one. Prayer and meditation are ways to connect with the Divine presence, just like talking to a friend or spending time with someone you care about."

"So, it's not about asking God for things?" Saharsha chimed in, his brow furrowed in thought.

"Not always, Saharsha," Dad replied. "While there's nothing wrong with asking for guidance or help, prayer and meditation can also be about expressing gratitude, offering love, or simply being present in the moment. It's a way to connect with something bigger than ourselves."

## THE LANGUAGE OF LOVE

Dad reached for a book on the shelf, its worn pages whispering tales of ancient wisdom. "Imagine the Divine as a loving parent," he said, opening the book. "Just like we love to spend time with our parents, the Divine might appreciate our devotion and love expressed through prayer and meditation."

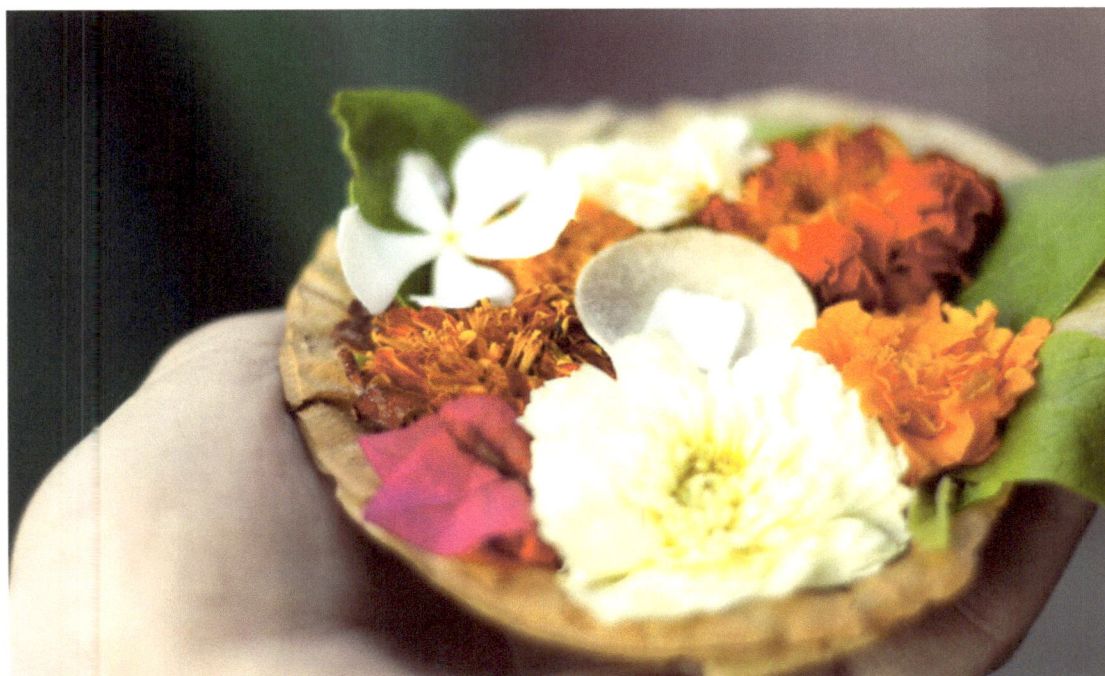

"But Dad," **Saumyaa** interjected, "Grandma also said there are different ways to worship. Can we choose how we want to connect with the Divine?"

Dad's eyes twinkled. "Absolutely, Saumyaa! There are many paths to the Divine, just like there are many ways to express love. Some people find comfort in focusing on a specific form of God, like Rama or Krishna. Others prefer a more formless approach, connecting with the Divine essence that flows through all things."

## THE STORY OF MIRA: A DEVOTEE'S DANCE

"There's a beautiful story about a princess named Mira," Dad began. "Mira was known for her deep devotion to Lord Krishna. She would sing and dance, expressing her love for him through music and movement. Mira loved Lord Krishna very much, even as a little girl. She felt his love all around her. Mira showed her love for Krishna in a special way — by dancing and singing! Every step and song was a way for her to tell Krishna how much she cared.

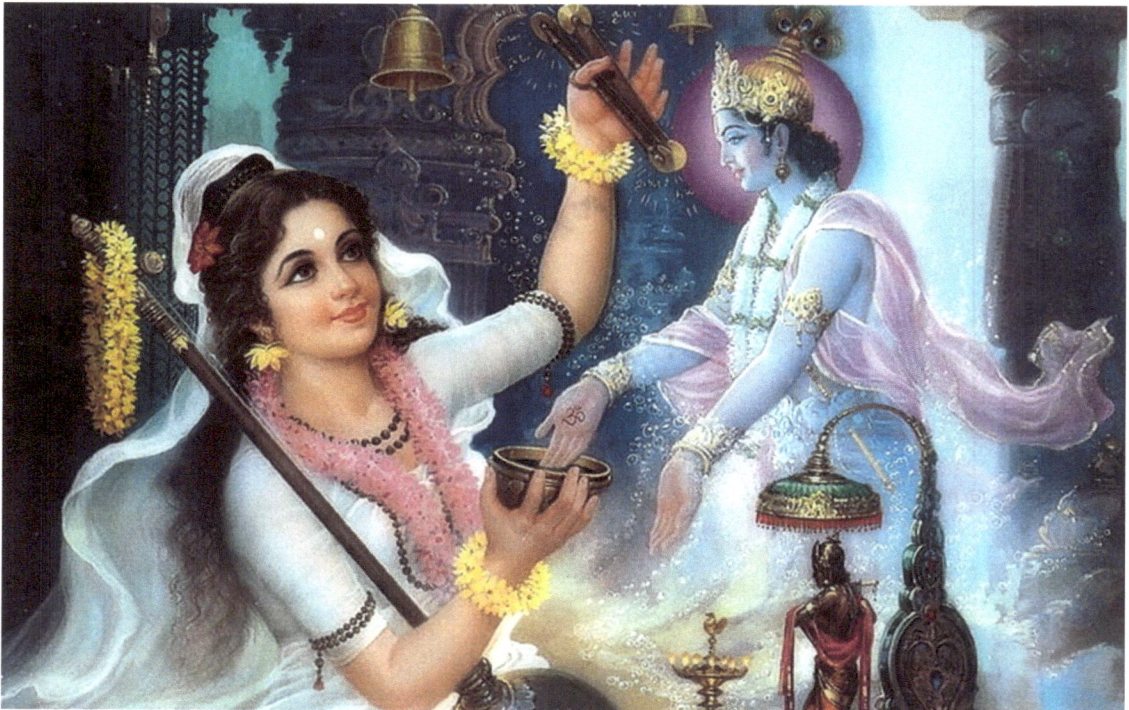

Some people thought princesses shouldn't dance and sing like that, but Mira didn't care. Her love for Krishna was more important than what others thought. She danced with all her heart, and it was beautiful!

Mira's dancing wasn't just fun, it was a way for her to connect with Krishna. It was like a special conversation between them, filled with love and joy. Even though others might not have understood, for Mira, her dancing was a sacred gift to Krishna, a celebration of their love.

When Dad finished the story, Saharsha and Saumyaa felt a sense of wonder. Mira's story showed them the power of love and devotion, and how it can take many different forms.

The fire crackled softly as Dad finished the story. Saharsha and Saumyaa sat in thoughtful silence for a moment.

SAHARSHA PONDERS: CAN ANIMALS FEEL THE DIVINE SPARK TOO?

"Do animals feel the Divine presence too, Dad? Even though they can't talk or pray?" Saharsha tilted his head, pondering the concept.

Dad's eyes crinkled with amusement. "An insightful question, Saharsha," he began. "Many traditions believe the Divine spark isn't exclusive to humans. Perhaps animals connect with the Divine in their own unique way, through the deep bond they share with nature and the instincts that guide them. Think about Lucky, for instance."

A smile spread across Dad's face. "Every time Lucky wags his tail so excitedly when you come home, or snuggles close to you for comfort, it could be his way of expressing his own kind of devotion. Maybe his playful spirit and his keen sense of smell, helping him navigate the world, are his way of experiencing the Divine in his own way."

He paused for a moment, a thoughtful expression gracing his face. "What you might be wondering, Saharsha," Dad continued, his voice gentle, "is if the love animals show their young, the loyalty they display, and the way their instincts contribute to the natural order – could these be their way of expressing their own connection to something greater? Lucky's love for you, his playful spirit, and his ability to follow a scent – all these things, in their own way, might be a reflection of the Divine spark that resides within him."

## PRAHLĀDA: A BEACON OF DEVOTION

"Dad," Saharsha finally spoke, "you mentioned devotion. Grandma told us about a boy named Prahlāda. Can you tell us his story?"

"Absolutely, Saharsha," Dad replied. "Prahlāda was the son of Hiranyakashipu, a powerful demon king. Hiranyakashipu, blinded by his arrogance, believed himself to be a god and demanded everyone worship him. Yet, Prahlada, even as a young boy (texts mention 5 years old), held onto his devotion to the true Divine, Lord Vishnu."

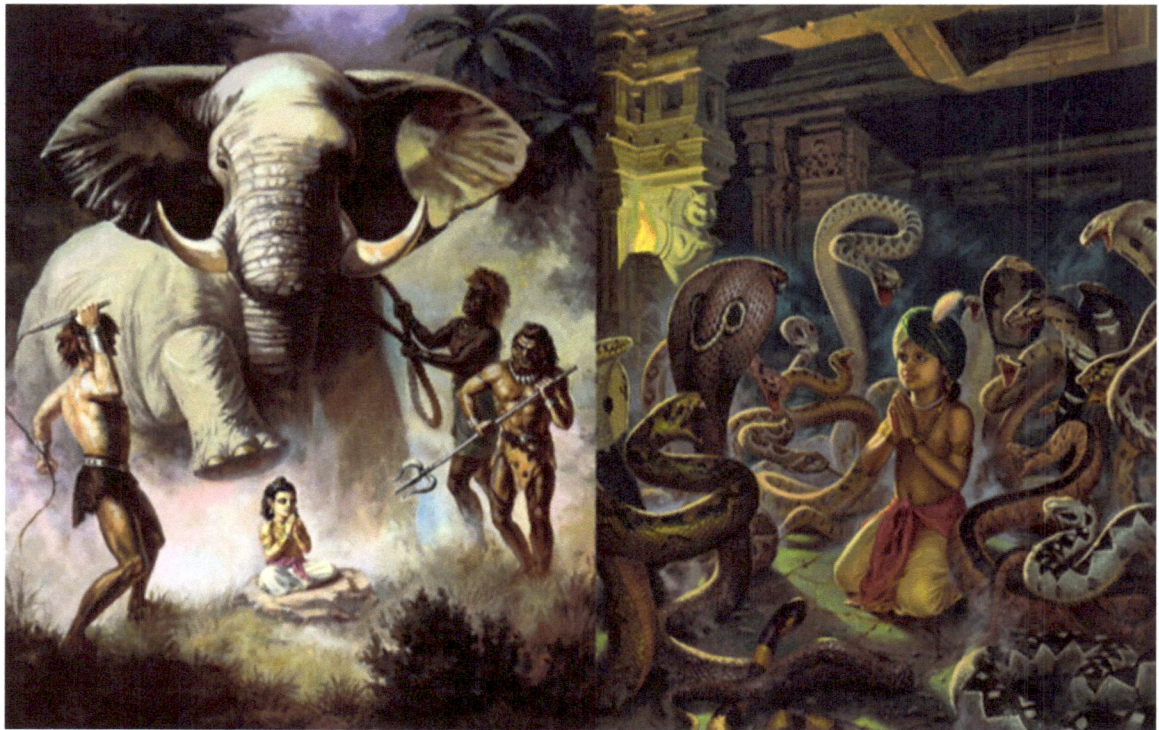

"But Dad, why didn't Prahlāda obey his father?" Saharsha asked.

Dad: "Prahlāda's faith in Lord Vishnu was unshakeable, Saharsha. He believed that true devotion should be directed towards the Supreme Being, not towards anyone else, even if it was his own father."

Saumyaa: "What happened when Prahlāda refused to worship his father?"

Dad: "Hiranyakashipu tried various ways to change Prahlāda's mind, but nothing worked. Finally, he ordered Prahlāda to be thrown into the ocean. However, Prahlāda's devotion protected him, and he emerged unharmed."

Saharsha: "Wow, that's incredible, Dad!"

Dad: "Indeed, Saharsha. Prahlāda's unwavering devotion touched Lord Vishnu's heart. When Prahlāda returned safely, his father demanded to see Vishnu. In response, Lord Vishnu appeared as Narasimha, a half-man, half-lion form, and vanquished Hiranyakashipu."

Saumyaa: "So, even as children, we can have deep devotion like Prahlāda?"

Dad: "Absolutely, Saumyaa. Prahlāda's story teaches us that age is not a barrier to devotion. Whether young or old, anyone can cultivate a loving relationship with the divine through devotion and faith."

From that night on, Saharsha and Saumyaa embarked on their own journeys of Bhakti. They experimented with different practices, from quiet meditation to singing hymns, always keeping their hearts open to the Divine presence that filled their world.

## CHAPTER SUMMARY: THE PATH OF LOVE (BHAKTI)

This chapter explores the concept of Bhakti, the path of devotional love for God. Dad explains that prayer and meditation are ways to connect with the Divine presence, not just asking for things.

Different Paths of Devotion:

- **Love as the Language:** Just like showing love to a parent, devotion can be expressed through prayer, meditation, or acts of love.

- **Choosing Your Way:** There's no single way to connect with the Divine. Some focus on a specific form of God, while others connect with a formless Divine essence.

## The Story of Mira:

Mira, a princess known for her deep devotion to Lord Krishna, expressed her love through singing and dancing. Despite societal disapproval, Mira's devotion remained pure and joyful, a unique way to connect with the Divine.

## Prahlāda: A Young Devotee

Dad shares the story of Prahlāda, a boy who remained devoted to Lord Vishnu even when his father, a powerful king, demanded he worship him instead. Prahlāda's unwavering faith protected him and showed that age is no barrier to devotion.

## Finding Your Own Path:

Inspired by these stories, **Saharsha** and **Saumyaa** embark on their own journeys of Bhakti, open to finding their own ways to connect with the Divine presence that surrounds them.

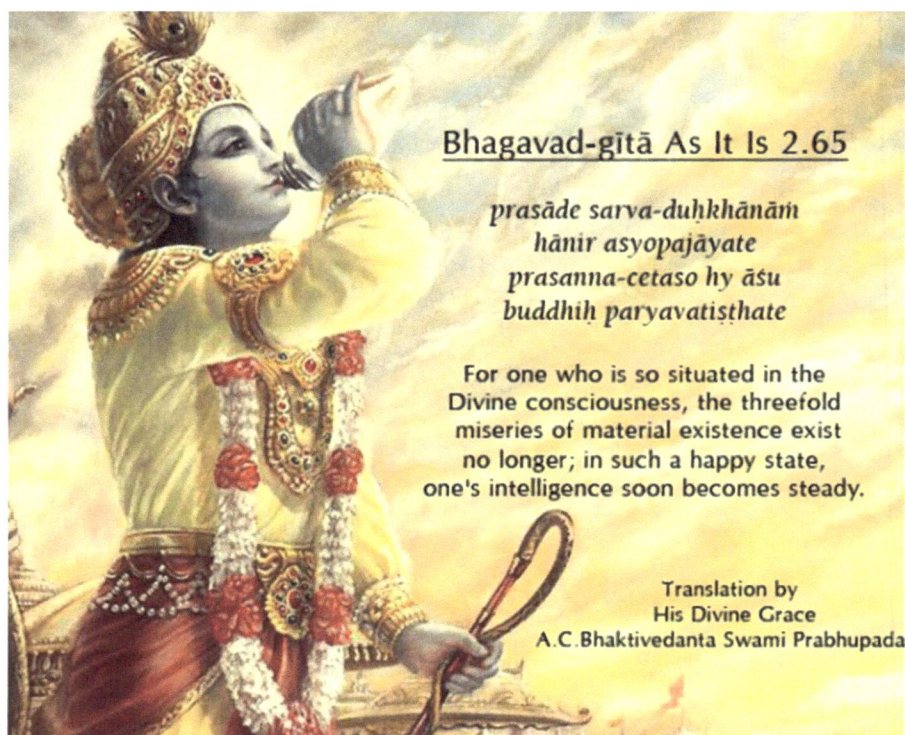

Bhagavad-gītā As It Is 2.65

*prasāde sarva-duḥkhānāṁ
hānir asyopajāyate
prasanna-cetaso hy āśu
buddhiḥ paryavatiṣṭhate*

For one who is so situated in the Divine consciousness, the threefold miseries of material existence exist no longer; in such a happy state, one's intelligence soon becomes steady.

Translation by
His Divine Grace
A.C.Bhaktivedanta Swami Prabhupada

# Chapter 13: Who Created Everything

## The Great Mystery

*The Great Mystery – Unveiling Origins*

*In the cloak of night, Saharsha and Saumyaa ponder the unfathomable: Who sculpted the heavens? With boundless curiosity and their father's wisdom as their guide, they plunge into the abyss of the cosmic unknown.*
*From the twinkling cosmos to the recesses of their very souls, mysteries beckon to be unraveled. Can they decipher the enigma that shrouds creation? Join them on a quest to unravel The Mystery Unveiled – Who Forged the Stars? Where answers ignite wonder and questions kindle the quest for truth.*

Saharsha lay sprawled on the soft grass, gazing up at the inky canvas of the night sky. A million stars twinkled like scattered diamonds, their light a silent conversation reaching across unimaginable distances. A sense of awe washed over him, a feeling that stretched from the tips of his toes to the very core of his being.

"Saumyaa, come look!" he called out, his voice a whisper against the vastness.

Saumyaa padded over, her bare feet brushing against the cool grass. She followed her brother's gaze, her eyes widening as they took in the celestial spectacle.

"Wow," she breathed, a single word carrying the weight of their shared wonder.

They lay in comfortable silence for a while, simply soaking in the beauty of the universe. Questions swirled in Saharsha's mind, each star a silent question mark.

"Saumyaa," he began hesitantly, "do you ever wonder who made all this?"

Saumyaa turned her head to look at him, her eyes reflecting the starlight. "Who made the stars, the moon, everything?" she echoed, her voice laced with curiosity.

A warm smile spread across Saharsha's face. He knew exactly who they should ask.

"Let's go find Dad," he declared, a newfound sense of purpose replacing his earlier awe.

**Together, hand-in-hand, they walked towards the house, hearts brimming with a child's innocent wonder, ready to embark on a journey to unravel the greatest mystery of all: the origin of everything.**

They pushed open the back door, the warm glow of the house spilling out to meet them like a comforting hug. Their Dad sat nestled in his favorite armchair, a book resting peacefully on his lap. He looked up as they entered, his eyes crinkling at the corners with a smile.

"There you two are," he said warmly, his voice a gentle rumble. "What brings you inside on such a beautiful night?"

Saharsha practically bounced on his toes. "Dad," he blurted out, unable to contain his excitement any longer, "we were looking at the stars, and Saumyaa and I were wondering..."

Saumyaa, more hesitant than her brother, chimed in, "Who made everything, Dad? The stars, the moon, the whole wide world?"

Dad chuckled softly. "Ah, the questions that have puzzled people for generations," he said, a thoughtful look replacing his smile momentarily. "Come, sit with me," he gestured, patting the space beside him on the armchair.

Saharsha and Saumyaa snuggled close, their anticipation building. Dad closed the book, placing it carefully on the side table.

"Well," he began, his voice taking on a storytelling quality, "tonight, we can explore the great mystery of creation. It's a story filled with wonder, faith, and maybe even a little bit of magic..."

Dad's voice trailed off, his eyes twinkling with amusement. He knew he had their full attention, and he was ready to embark on a journey of discovery with them.

Dad smiled warmly at Saharsha and Saumyaa as they gathered around him, their eyes gleaming with curiosity. "Dad, how does our body know how to do so many things?" Saharsha asked, his brow furrowed in thought.

"That's a great question, Saharsha," Dad replied warmly. "Our bodies are truly remarkable. They're made up of five basic elements - earth, water, fire, air, and ether. These elements work together to give us the ability to eat, sleep, think, talk, walk, run, and so much more."

"But how does our body know how to do all that?" Saumyaa chimed in, her eyes wide with wonder.

"Well, Saumyaa, inside our bodies, there's something called the Spirit or Atman," Dad explained. "It's like a special power source that gives us the energy to do all these things. This spark of life within us might be a reflection of the greater Divine force that created everything." "But who created the Spirit and the whole universe?"

Saharsha asked, his curiosity piqued. Dad paused, considering Saharsha's question thoughtfully. "That's a big question, Saharsha. Many people believe there's a creator behind everything in the universe. Just like how someone made the cars we drive and the houses we live in, there's a divine force that created the sun, the earth, the moon, and the stars  We call that force God or the creator."

"But then, who created God?" Saumyaa asked, her brow creased in confusion.

Dad smiled gently. "That's a question people have pondered for centuries, Saumyaa. The truth is, God has always existed and will always exist. He's the origin of everything, but He Himself has no origin. It's like trying to imagine the beginning of time itself − it's beyond our human understanding."

"Can we see God, Dad?" Saharsha inquired, his eyes wide with curiosity.

Dad shook his head. "God is beyond what our eyes can see, Saharsha. He's everywhere, present in all things, yet not limited by a physical body like us. Imagine the vastness of the universe, with billions of stars and galaxies. God's presence is like that – immense and all-encompassing."

"But then, how can we know and understand God?" Saumyaa asked, her mind buzzing with questions.

Dad smiled warmly at his children. "We can't know God through our minds or intellect alone, Saumyaa. We can only know Him through faith, belief, and Self-knowledge. When we understand that the same divine spark exists within all living things, from the tiniest insect to the highest mountain, we learn to treat everyone and everything with kindness and respect."

"Wow, that's amazing," Saharsha exclaimed, his mind spinning with new ideas.

"Yes, it is," Dad agreed. "And just like how we can't fully describe the depth of the ocean, we can't fully describe the greatness of God. He's beyond our understanding, but we can feel His presence in the beauty and wonder of the world around us. The sunrise, the twinkling stars, the love we share with each other – these are all glimpses of the Divine."

As Saharsha and Saumyaa listened intently to their dad's words, their hearts filled with a sense of wonder and awe at the vastness of the universe and the mysteries of creation.

"Hey, Dad, can you tell us a story about someone who tried to understand God?" Saharsha asked eagerly.

Dad smiled, knowing just the story to captivate his children's imaginations and deepen their understanding of the divine.

"Of course, Saharsha," Dad replied. "Let me tell you the story of a Firefly."

# THE STORY OF THE CURIOUS FIREFLY

Once upon a time, in a bustling forest filled with life, lived a tiny firefly named Flicker. Unlike other fireflies, Flicker wasn't content with simply lighting up the night sky. He yearned for a deeper understanding of the source of his own light.

"Why do I glow?" Flicker would ask his friends, blinking his tiny beacon.

"It's just what fireflies do," they would reply, content with their simple existence.

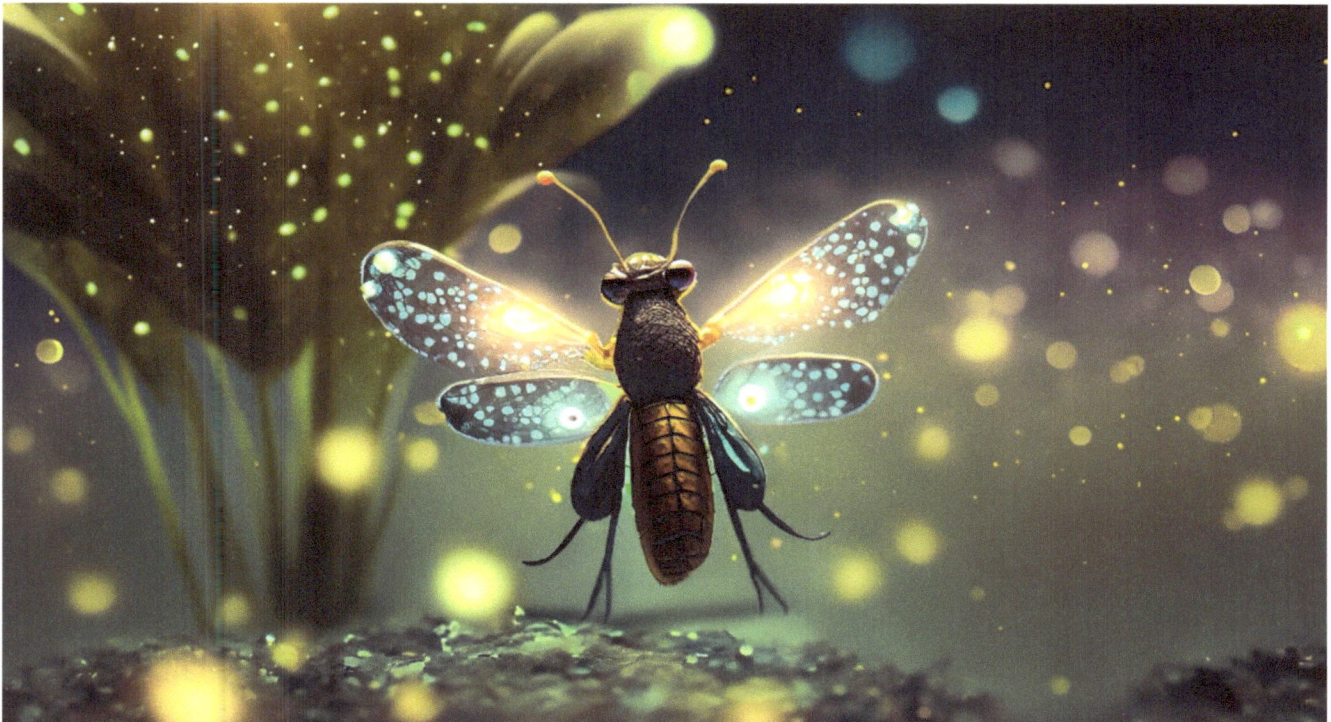

But Flicker wasn't satisfied. He embarked on a journey, flitting from flower to flower, asking every creature he met about the source of light. The wise old owl hooted about the sun, the mighty oak whispered about the moon, but none could explain Flicker's own inner glow.

Disheartened, Flicker perched on a blade of grass, ready to give up. Suddenly, a gentle voice filled the air. "Little one, why the long face?"

Flicker looked up to see a beautiful butterfly, its wings shimmering with an otherworldly light. He explained his quest to understand his own light.

The butterfly smiled. "Your light, dear Flicker, comes from a spark within you, a tiny piece of the Great Light that shines in all things."

Flicker tilted his head. "The Great Light?"

"Yes," the butterfly explained. "It's the source of all creation, the force that makes the sun rise and the stars twinkle. It's the same light that makes you glow, little firefly."

Flicker pondered this for a moment. "So, the Great Light is everywhere?"

"Yes," the butterfly replied, "It's in the warmth of the sun, the gentle breeze, and the love shared between friends."

Suddenly, Flicker understood. His own light wasn't just about illuminating the night; it was a part of something much bigger, a connection to the Great Light that shone in everything around him.

From that day on, Flicker no longer just blinked his light. He used it to illuminate the path for lost beetles, to guide moths to blooming flowers, and to share his joy with the other fireflies. He understood that his own light, though small, was a reflection of the Great Light that connected him to the entire universe.

As Dad finished the story of the curious firefly, Saharsha and Saumyaa sat mesmerized.

"Wow," Saharsha breathed, "so even a tiny firefly has a connection to something so big?"

Dad chuckled. "Exactly, Saharsha. The story reminds us that even though we may seem small in this vast universe, we all carry a spark of the Divine within us. This spark might be the very essence that gave rise to all creation."

Saumyaa's brow furrowed in thought. "So, the Great Light isn't just a source of kindness, but maybe the source of everything – the stars, the moon, even us?"

"That's a very insightful question, Saumyaa," Dad replied warmly. "Many people believe the Great Light, or God, is the ultimate creator, the force behind the universe and all that exists. While we may not fully understand how it all happened, the wonder and beauty around us point to something grander than ourselves."

Saharsha and Saumyaa sat in comfortable silence for a moment, contemplating this new understanding. The night sky outside seemed to shimmer with a renewed sense of mystery and awe.

"Thanks, Dad," Saharsha finally said, a genuine smile spreading across his face. "That story and explanation were amazing."

Dad ruffled Saharsha's hair playfully. "You're welcome, son. Remember, the next time you see a firefly blinking in the darkness, think of Flicker and the Great Light that connects us all, the very same light that might hold the secrets of creation."

With hearts brimming with curiosity and a renewed sense of wonder about the universe, Saharsha and Saumyaa snuggled closer to their Dad, ready to drift off to sleep under the watchful gaze of the stars, each twinkling with a tiny spark of the Divine mystery.

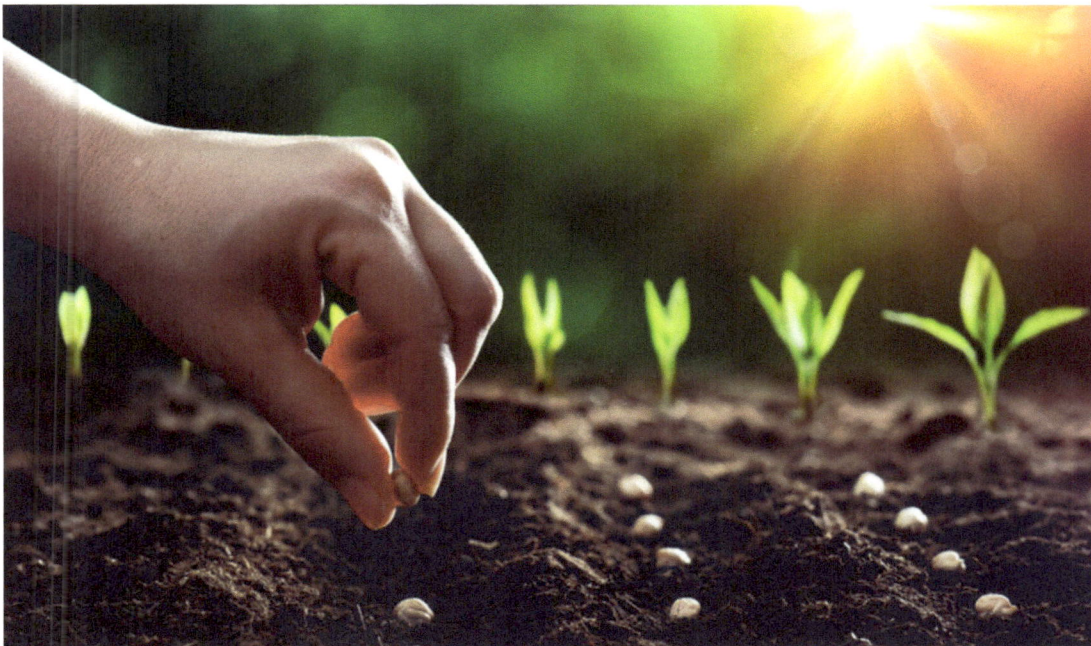

## CHAPTER SUMMARY: WHO CREATED EVERYTHING? – A SPARK OF WONDER

Saharsha and Saumyaa, filled with curiosity, ask their Dad about the marvels of their bodies and the vast universe. Dad explains how our bodies, composed of five elements, are powered by a life force called the Spirit or Atman, similar to the concept of **Atman** explored in the Bhagavad Gita, the eternal essence within all living beings.

This exploration leads to a bigger question: **who created everything?** Dad introduces the **concept of God**, a divine force many believe is behind all creation. Just as Krishna, in the Bhagavad Gita, speaks of a higher power, this force might have created the universe. However, God's existence transcends our complete understanding.

**Unveiling the Divine:** We can't see God with our physical eyes, yet He's present everywhere. He doesn't have a physical form but possesses the ability to perceive everything, similar to how Krishna describes the omnipresence of the divine in the Bhagavad Gita.

**Connecting with the Divine:** Understanding God isn't solely intellectual. Faith, belief, and self-knowledge are crucial for fostering a connection with the divine spark within us all, just as the Bhagavad Gita emphasizes the importance of Bhakti (devotion) and Jnana (knowledge) in seeking the divine.

**The Spark of Creation:** The chapter delves into the connection between the Creator and creation. Some believe God is like the sun, with everything bathed in His light, a part of His being. This concept resonates with the Bhagavad Gita's portrayal of the divine as the source of all creation.

The chapter concludes with a sense of awe at the universe's vastness and the mystery of creation. While we might not fully grasp God, we can feel His presence in the beauty and wonder surrounding us. This spark of wonder ignites a desire to explore further, leaving Saharsha and Saumyaa with a thirst for knowledge about the divine, inspiring them to delve deeper into the wisdom of the Bhagavad Gita.

# Chapter 14: The Nature's Three Gears

"

## *3 Gunas: Unraveling the Tug-of-War Within*

*As Saharsha and Saumyaa bask in the warmth of a lazy afternoon, their innocent play is interrupted by a profound inquiry:*
*Why do our moods ebb and flow? Through their father's guidance and the Bhagavad Gita's wisdom, they explore the Nature's Three Gears – the subtle forces shaping human behavior. Can they tame the gears of Goodness, Passion, and Laziness to navigate life's complexities? Join them on a journey of self-discovery where the secrets of the human spirit await revelation.*

## THE TUG-OF-WAR WITHIN

The afternoon sun cast long shadows across the backyard as Saharsha and

Saumyaa chased each other through the sprinkler, shrieking with delight. Their laughter echoed through the air, a symphony of pure joy. Suddenly, Saharsha skidded to a stop, his chest heaving with exertion.

"Wow, I'm beat!" he declared, collapsing onto the soft grass.

Saumyaa, a few steps behind, mirrored his actions, panting slightly. "Me too," she agreed, wiping a stray droplet of water from her forehead.

A comfortable silence settled between them as they watched fat raindrops plop onto the thirsty earth. Saharsha, never one for quiet contemplation for too long, broke the silence.

"Dad!" he called out, his voice laced with curiosity. "Why do I sometimes feel like I can run forever, but other times I just want to lie in bed and do nothing?"

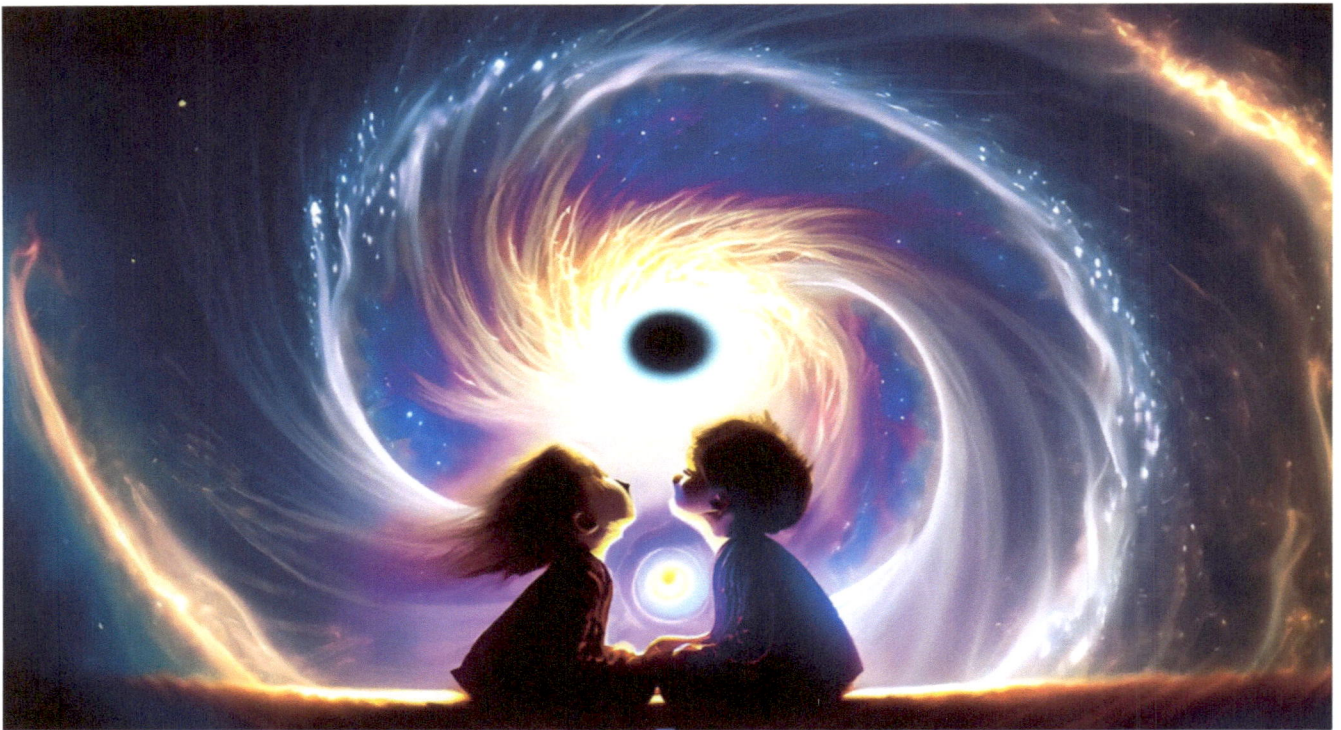

Saumyaa tilted her head, her brow furrowed in thought. "Yeah, Dad," she chimed in, "sometimes I feel super focused and can finish all my homework in a flash, but other days it takes forever, and I get distracted easily."

Dad, who had been observing their playful exchange from the porch swing, chuckled warmly. He knew his children well, and their questions reflected a deeper curiosity about the world and themselves. Rising from the swing, he walked towards them, his smile radiating warmth.

"Those are great questions, Saharsha and Saumyaa," he began. "Have you ever heard of something called the Gunas?"

Dad smiled, knowing it was time to unravel the mysteries of nature for his eager children. "Well, Saumyaa," he began, "the world around us, and even ourselves, are influenced by three different forces, or Gunas. These are like different gears that determine how we feel and act, a concept we find explored in the Bhagavad Gita."

Imagine nature as a giant machine, Dad said. These Gunas are like three different gears that control our actions and feelings.

| Tamas | Sattva | Rajas |
|---|---|---|
| Dull mind | Clear, calm mind | Energetic mind |
| Obscures Awareness | Reveals Awareness | Distorts Awareness |
| Veiling power | Revealing power | Projecting power |
| Apathetic, lazy, sluggish, foggy, heaviness, prone to depression | Easy-going, balanced, peaceful, harmonious, contented | Busy, passionate, aggressive, frustrated, excited, prone to anxiety |
| Fear / Avoidance | Truth / Beingness | Desire / Anxiety |
| Allows for rest and sleep | Allows for discernment | Allows for motivation |
| Hinders Self-inquiry & meditation | Facilitates Self-inquiry & meditation | Hinders Self-inquiry & meditation |

- **The Goodness Gear (Sattva):** When we're in the goodness gear, we feel happy and peaceful. We want to help others, learn new things, and make good choices.

- **The Passion Gear (Rajas):** This gear makes us crave excitement and new things. We might work hard to get something we want, but sometimes this gear can make us greedy or selfish.

- **The Laziness Gear (Tamas):** When we're in this gear, we feel sluggish and uninterested in anything. We might make bad choices or neglect our responsibilities.

Dad explained that everyone experiences all three Gunas throughout the day. Sometimes, one gear might be stronger than the others. The important thing is to be aware of these forces and try to stay in the goodness gear as much as possible.

"So, can we control these gears, Dad?" Saumyaa asked.

Dad smiled. "We can't directly control them, Saumyaa, but we can influence them with our choices. By helping others, being honest, and learning good things, we can stay in the goodness gear more often."

"And what happens if we stay in the goodness gear all the time?" Saharsha wondered.

Saumyaa wrinkled her nose in thought. "So, these modes control how we feel and act?"

"Exactly," Dad nodded. "But it's up to us to choose which mode we want to be in."

"But how do we choose?" Saharsha asked, his brow furrowed.

"We can rise above these modes by making good choices and practicing devotion to God," Dad replied. "When we serve others with love and kindness, we rise above the influence of the Gunas and become closer to God."

"That sounds hard," Saumyaa said softly.

"It can be," Dad agreed. "But with effort and devotion, anything is possible."

"Hey, Dad, can you tell us a story to help us understand better?" Saharsha asked eagerly.

Dad smiled, knowing just the story to illustrate the nature of the Gunas.

"One sunny day, a farmer set out to tend to his fields," Dad began. "As he walked, he came across three different types of soil. The first soil was rich, fertile, and well-nourished by the sun and rain. The second soil was dry, barren, and devoid of nutrients. And the third soil was somewhere in between, with patches of fertility amidst barrenness."

Saharsha and Saumyaa listened intently, their imaginations conjuring images of the farmer and his fields.

"The farmer planted seeds in each type of soil," Dad continued. "In the fertile soil, the seeds sprouted quickly, growing into healthy, robust plants. In the barren soil, the seeds struggled to take root, withering away before they could flourish. And in the soil with patches of fertility, the seeds grew sporadically, their growth hindered by the surrounding barrenness."

"So, what happened next?" Saharsha asked eagerly.

"The farmer realized that the quality of the soil determined the success of the seeds," Dad explained. "Similarly, in our lives, the three Gunas—Sattva, Rajas, and Tamas—affect our growth and development. When we cultivate qualities of goodness, purity, and clarity (Sattva), we create fertile ground for our potential to blossom. But when we're consumed by desires, ambitions, and distractions (Rajas), our growth is stunted, like seeds struggling in barren soil. And when we're plagued by laziness, ignorance, and darkness (Tamas), our potential remains untapped, buried beneath layers of inertia and apathy."

Saumyaa nodded in understanding. "So, just like the farmer tended to his soil, we must tend to our minds and hearts, nurturing qualities that uplift and inspire."

"Exactly," Dad affirmed with a smile. "By cultivating Sattva—goodness, purity, and clarity—we create the optimal conditions for our growth and evolution. We become like the fertile soil, fertile ground for our dreams, aspirations, and spiritual aspirations to take root and flourish."

As Saharsha and Saumyaa absorbed the wisdom of the story, they felt inspired to tend to the soil of their own hearts, nurturing qualities of goodness, purity, and clarity in their daily lives.

"Saharsha, Saumyaa, always remember that the choices we make and the actions we take shape the soil of our hearts," Dad continued. "Just as the farmer tended to his fields, we must tend to our minds and spirits, cultivating qualities that uplift and inspire us."

Saharsha nodded thoughtfully. "So, by focusing on goodness and purity, we can create fertile ground for our dreams and aspirations to grow."

"Exactly," Dad replied, his eyes twinkling with pride at his children's understanding. "And just as the farmer nurtured his soil with care and attention, we must nurture our hearts with love, compassion, and wisdom."

Saumyaa chimed in, her voice filled with determination. "We'll make sure to cultivate the soil of our hearts every day, Dad, so that we can grow into the best versions of ourselves."

Dad smiled warmly at his children. "I have no doubt that you will, my dear ones. With each act of kindness, each moment of self-reflection, and each step towards personal growth, you'll be tending to the soil of your hearts and nurturing the seeds of greatness within you."

As Saharsha and Saumyaa embraced their father's words, they felt a renewed sense of purpose and direction. With hearts full of determination and minds filled with wisdom, they embarked on their journey of self-discovery, knowing that they held the power to cultivate a future filled with joy, fulfillment, and abundance.

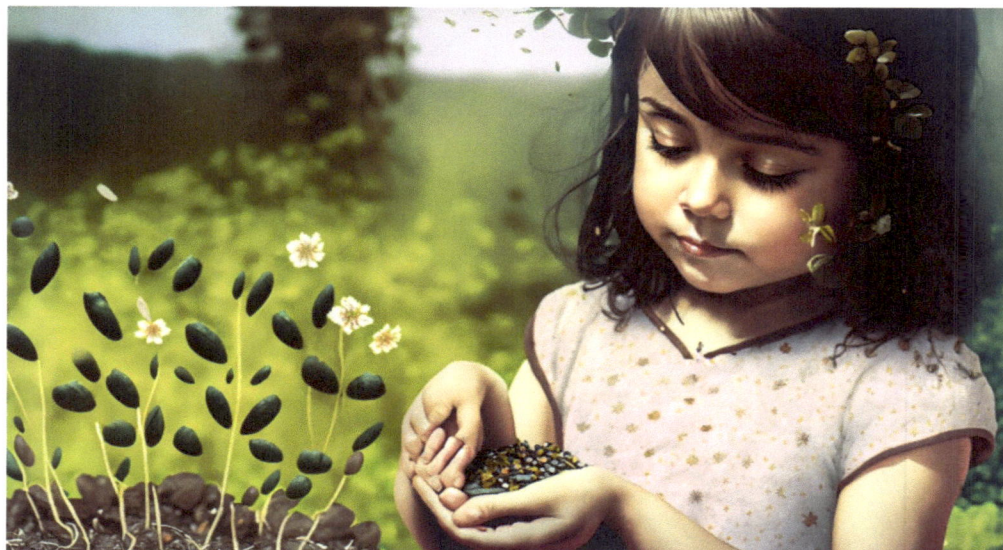

## CHAPTER SUMMARY: NATURE'S GEARS

This chapter delves into the fascinating concept of Gunas, a trio of natural forces explored in the Bhagavad Gita, a holy book filled with wisdom. These Gunas, like gears in a grand machine, influence our actions and feelings throughout the day.

Imagine your body and mind as a machine, Saharsha and Saumyaa. The Gunas act as three different gears that control your energy levels and motivations.

1. **Sattva (Goodness Gear):** Inspires happiness, peace, and helpfulness. It sparks curiosity, good decision-making, and positive contributions.

2. **Rajas (Passion Gear):** Ignites excitement and motivation for new experiences and goals. Yet, it can veer into selfishness and greed if uncontrolled.

3. **Tamas (Laziness Gear):** Induces sluggishness and lack of motivation, potentially clouding judgment and fostering neglect of responsibilities.

The chapter explains that we experience all three Gunas throughout the day. Sometimes, the goodness gear might be driving your actions, while other times, the passion or laziness gear might be more dominant.

The key message of the chapter is to strive to stay in the goodness gear as much as possible. By making good choices, helping others, and cultivating positive qualities, you can strengthen the influence of Sattva in your life.

The chapter also introduces the concept of liberation, a state beyond the influence of the Gunas. In this state, you experience true peace and freedom. It can be attained through devotion to a higher power and by practicing self-discipline.

This exploration of the Gunas equips Saharsha and Saumyaa with tools to understand their own motivations and make conscious choices. As they learn to navigate these gears, they move closer to a life filled with purpose, joy, and inner peace.

# Chapter 15: The Supreme Being and Beyond

"

### *Unraveling the Cosmos*

*Beyond the dance of light and shadow lies a realm of boundless wonder. Saharsha and Saumyaa, fueled by their thirst for knowledge, embark on a journey deeper than they ever imagined. Questions blossom like petals in their minds, leading them to the heart of existence. With their father as their guide, they venture into the realm of the Supreme Being. As they unravel the mysteries of the universe, they discover a connection that transcends time and space. Join them on this awe-inspiring quest to unlock the secrets of the cosmos and glimpse the divine beyond the gears.*

## A GLIMPSE BEYOND THE GEARS

The dappled sunlight filtering through the leaves cast a mesmerizing dance of light and shadow on the grass. Saharsha and Saumyaa, their curiosity piqued by their recent exploration of the Gunas, sat nestled beside their Dad, eager to delve deeper into the mysteries of the universe.

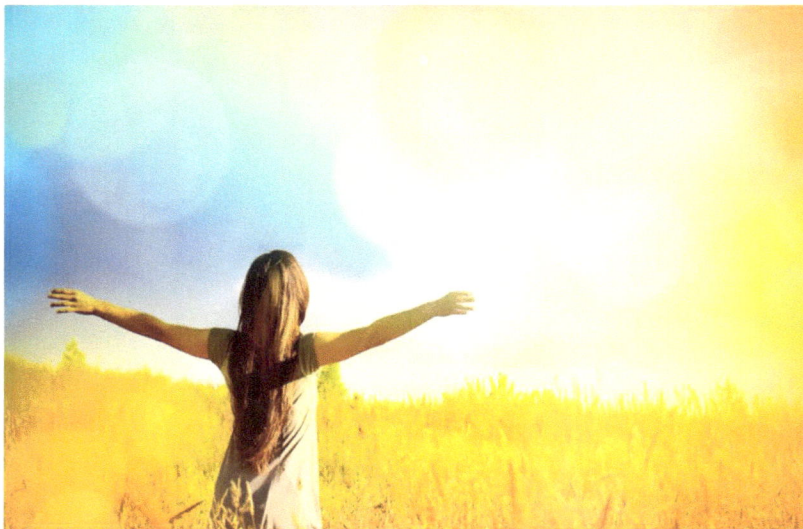

"Dad," Saharsha began, his voice brimming with inquisitiveness, "last time we learned about the Gunas, these natural forces that influence how we feel and act. But is there something beyond them? Something that controls these gears themselves?"

Saumyaa, ever the thoughtful one, chimed in, "Yes, Dad. We understood that staying in the goodness gear (Sattva) is important. But who or what makes Sattva, Rajas, and Tamas exist in the first place?"

Dad smiled warmly, his eyes twinkling with delight at their insatiable curiosity. "Excellent questions, Saharsha and Saumyaa," he replied. "You've reached a fascinating juncture in your exploration. Today, we'll explore the concept of the Supreme Being, the ultimate source of everything, the force that sets the very gears of nature in motion."

Leaning closer, he continued, "Imagine the universe as a vast, intricate machine, Saharsha. The Gunas, like we discussed, are the gears that keep it functioning. But there must be an engineer, a master mechanic, who designed and built this machine, wouldn't you agree?"

Saharsha and Saumyaa exchanged a thoughtful glance, their minds grappling with this new concept. The idea of a supreme being, a force beyond the Gunas, sparked a sense of awe and wonder within them.

"That's right," Dad confirmed, his voice filled with reverence. "In the Bhagavad Gita, and in many other spiritual traditions, this supreme being is referred to by different names – Brahman, the Absolute, or Paramatma, the Supreme Self. It's the source of all creation the essence of everything that exists."

With rapt attention, Saharsha and Saumyaa leaned in further, eager to unravel the mysteries of the Supreme Being and its connection to the world around them, their journey of self-discovery taking an exciting new turn.

Saharsha and Saumyaa listened intently as Dad explained the intricate concepts of the Supreme Spirit, Spirit, Divine Beings, and individual souls.

"The Supreme Spirit, also known as the Supreme Person or the Absolute, is the ultimate source of everything," Dad began. "It's like the root of a tree, providing nourishment and support to everything else."

Saumyaa nodded, absorbing the information. "And Spirit, or Brahma, is a part of the Supreme Spirit, like the trunk of the tree," she summarized.

"Exactly," Dad affirmed. "And Divine Beings, such as Vishnu, Brahma, and Mahesha, are expansions of Spirit. They play important roles in the functioning of the cosmos."

Saharsha raised an eyebrow. "But what about individual souls? Are they also part of Divine Beings?"

Dad smiled at his curious children. "No, individual souls, or Jiva, are distinct entities. They're like the fruits and flowers of the tree, separate from Divine Beings but still connected to the Supreme Spirit. As an old proverb says, 'The sun shines on all, but only a mirror reflects its light.'" The Supreme Spirit shines on all creation, but individual souls have the potential to reflect that divine light through their thoughts and actions.

Saumyaa pondered for a moment. "So, everything in the universe, from planets to living beings, is interconnected and part of the Supreme Being?"

"Exactly," Dad affirmed. "Even the planets, like the Sun and the Moon, are creations of Divine Beings and ultimately connected to the Supreme Spirit. Another proverb says, 'Three things cannot be long hidden: the sun, the moon, and the truth.' The Supreme Spirit, like the sun, may be beyond our immediate perception, but its truth is always present."

"Wow," Saharsha exclaimed, "it's incredible to think about the vastness and interconnectedness of everything!"

Dad chuckled. "Indeed, it's a wonder to contemplate. And speaking of wonders, let me tell you a story about Baby Krishna, who embodied the essence of the Supreme Spirit."

Saumyaa and Saharsha leaned in eagerly as Dad began recounting the tale of Krishna's playful antics and divine revelation to his mother, Yashoda.

"And just as Baby Krishna brought joy and wonder to those around him," Dad concluded, "so too does the Supreme Spirit infuse our lives with meaning and purpose."

As Saharsha and Saumyaa reflected on the story and Dad's words, they felt a deep sense of connection to something greater than themselves, a universal force that bound all of creation together in harmony and love.

Dad smiled warmly at Saharsha and Saumyaa's thoughtful expressions. "That's a great way to put it," he said. "And just like a tree has different parts, like the roots, trunk, branches, leaves, and fruits, our universe also has different aspects, all connected to the Supreme Spirit."

Saumyaa, her curiosity piqued, asked, "But how do we know all this? Can we see the Supreme Spirit?"

"Well, Saumyaa," Dad replied, "the Supreme Spirit is beyond our physical senses. We can't see, touch, or hear the Supreme Spirit like we do with everyday objects. It's something we understand through faith, intuition, and spiritual wisdom."

"So, to understand the Supreme Spirit, we often use analogies and stories," Dad continued. "For instance, let me tell you the story of baby Krishna."

Saumyaa and Saharsha nodded eagerly, their interest piqued.

Dad launched into the tale of Baby Krishna's playful antics and divine revelation to his mother, Yashoda, illustrating how the Supreme Spirit pervades everything in the universe, yet remains beyond our physical perception.

"Wow, that's amazing!" Saharsha exclaimed when Dad finished the story.

"Indeed, it is," Dad agreed. "And just like Krishna, the Supreme Spirit is both immanent, meaning present within everything, and transcendent, existing beyond the material world."

"But how can we connect with the Supreme Spirit if we can't see or touch Him?" Saumyaa asked, her brow furrowed in thought.

"That's where spirituality comes in," Dad explained. "Through practices like prayer, meditation, and selfless service, we can cultivate a deeper connection with the Supreme Spirit. It's not about seeing with our eyes but feeling with our hearts."

Saumyaa nodded in understanding. "Thank you for explaining, Dad."

"You're welcome, Saumyaa," Dad replied with a gentle smile. "Remember, the journey to understand the Supreme Spirit is a lifelong one, filled with wonder and discovery."

As Dad observed Saharsha and Saumyaa absorbing the profound concepts, he felt a sense of pride in their inquisitive minds and eagerness to learn. Encouraged by their interest, he continued to impart wisdom.

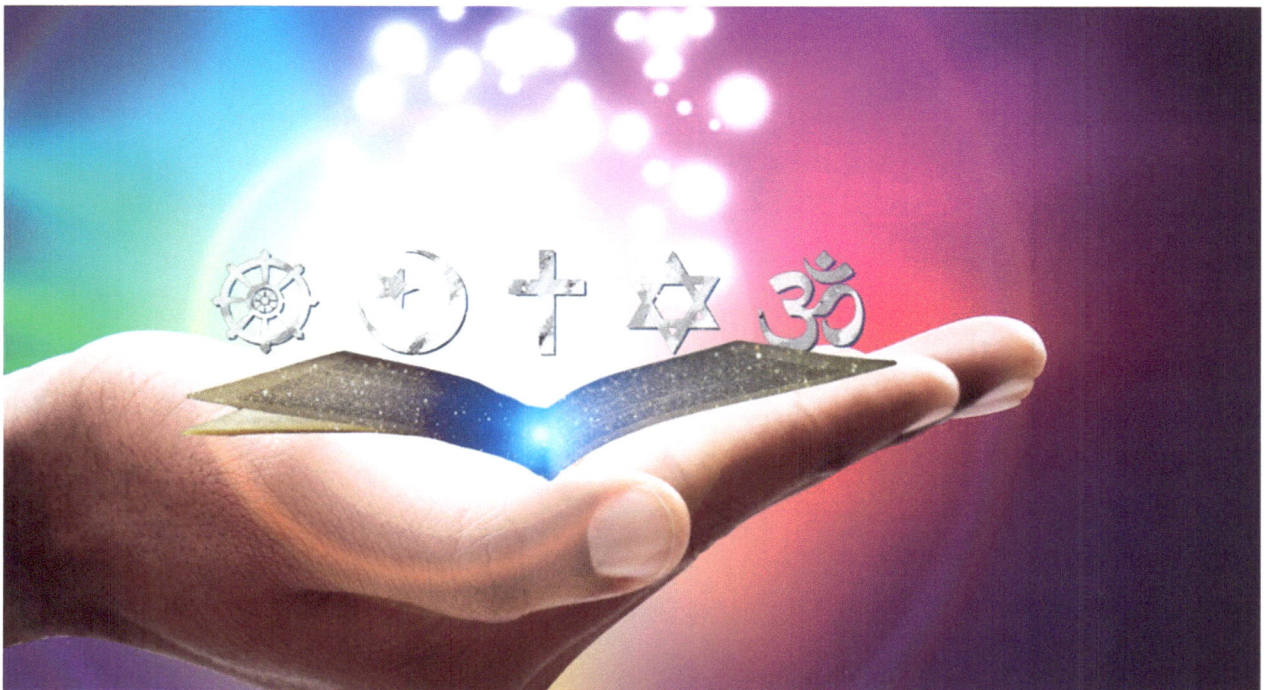

"Think of the Supreme Spirit like the sun," Dad began, gesturing toward the window where the afternoon sunlight streamed in. "We can't look directly at the sun because its brilliance would blind us. Similarly, the Supreme Spirit's radiance is so vast and powerful that our limited senses cannot fully comprehend it."

Saumyaa and Saharsha nodded, understanding the analogy.

"But just because we can't see the sun doesn't mean we can't feel its warmth or see its effects," Dad continued. "In the same way, although we can't perceive the Supreme Spirit with our physical senses, we can experience its presence through the beauty of nature, the kindness of others, and the love in our hearts."

Saharsha raised a hand, a question forming in his mind. "Dad, if the Supreme Spirit is everywhere, does that mean it's also inside us?"

Dad nodded, acknowledging the insightful question. "Yes, Saharsha. The Supreme Spirit dwells within each of us as the spark of divinity. It's like a tiny flame that illuminates our souls and guides us on our spiritual journey."

Saumyaa's eyes widened with curiosity. "But if the Supreme Spirit is within us, why do we sometimes feel disconnected or lost?"

Dad paused, considering Saumyaa's question thoughtfully. "That's because our minds often become clouded by distractions, desires, and doubts," he explained. "We forget our divine nature and get caught up in the illusions of the material world. But through spiritual practices like meditation, self-reflection, and prayer, we can clear away the fog and rediscover our connection to the Supreme Spirit."

Saumyaa and Saharsha listened attentively, absorbing Dad's words like sponges.

"In essence," Dad concluded, "our journey is not about seeking something external, but rather uncovering the eternal truth that lies within us. It's a journey of self-discovery and awakening to the presence of the Supreme Spirit in every aspect of our lives."

As the conversation drew to a close, Saharsha and Saumyaa felt a newfound sense of clarity and purpose. With Dad's guidance, they embarked on their own spiritual journey, eager to explore the depths of their souls and connect with the boundless expanse of the Supreme Spirit.

## CHAPTER SUMMARY: THE SUPREME BEING AND BEYOND

This chapter explores the concept of the Supreme Spirit, divine beings, and individual souls from a spiritual perspective.

- **The Supreme Spirit:** Dad explains the Supreme Spirit as the ultimate source of everything, like the root of a tree nourishing everything else. Saumyaa adds that it connects everything in the universe.

- **Spirit and Divine Beings:** Spirit (Brahma) is a part of the Supreme Spirit, while Divine Beings like Vishnu, Brahma, and Mahesh are expansions of Spirit with specific roles.

- **Individual Souls:** Jivas, or individual souls, are distinct entities connected to the Supreme Spirit but separate from Divine Beings, like fruits and flowers of the tree.

- **Stories and Analogies:** Dad uses the story of Krishna to illustrate the Supreme Spirit's essence.

Key Points:

- The Supreme Spirit is beyond physical senses and is understood through faith, intuition, and spiritual wisdom.

- The universe has different aspects, all connected to the Supreme Spirit.

- We can connect with the Supreme Spirit through practices like prayer, meditation, and service.

- The Supreme Spirit is both immanent (present within everything) and transcendent (existing beyond the material world).

# Chapter 16: Divine Light vs. Demonic Darkness

## *Dive into the Depths*

*Embark on a journey into the heart of human nature as Saumyaa's curiosity sparks a profound exploration. Join her and Saharsha as they unravel the dichotomy between divine light and demonic darkness, guided by their wise father's teachings. Discover the two forces that shape our choices and actions, leading us down paths of goodness or turmoil. Through captivating stories like "The Dog and the Bone" and "Queen Draupadi," learn the invaluable lessons of cultivating virtues and overcoming vices. Prepare to be inspired to cultivate your inner garden of goodness and illuminate the world with the light of the Bhaaavad Gita.*

## The Seed of Curiosity

Saumyaa's brow furrowed in concentration as she observed the world around her. "Dad," she began, her voice brimming with curiosity, "why do some people seem kind and helpful, while others are mean and selfish?"

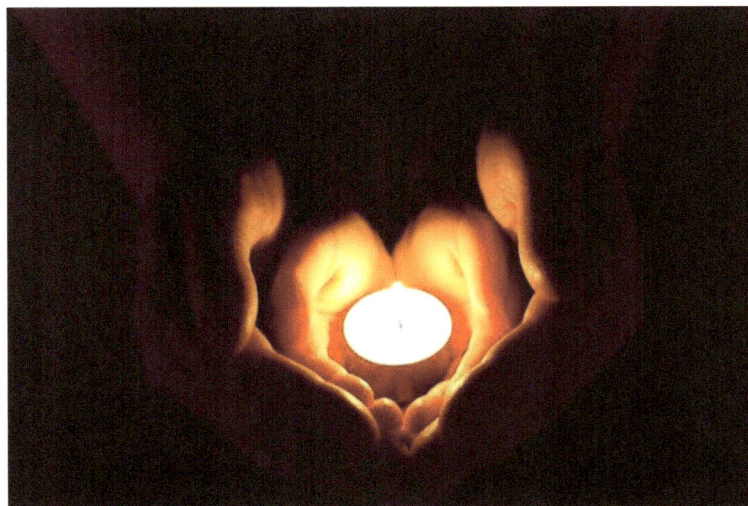

Dad, ever patient and insightful, smiled warmly. "That's a great question, Saumyaa," he replied. 'The way people behave depends on the qualities they possess, like different colored threads woven into the fabric of their character."

## THE TWO PATHS: DIVINE LIGHT AND DEMONIC DARKNESS

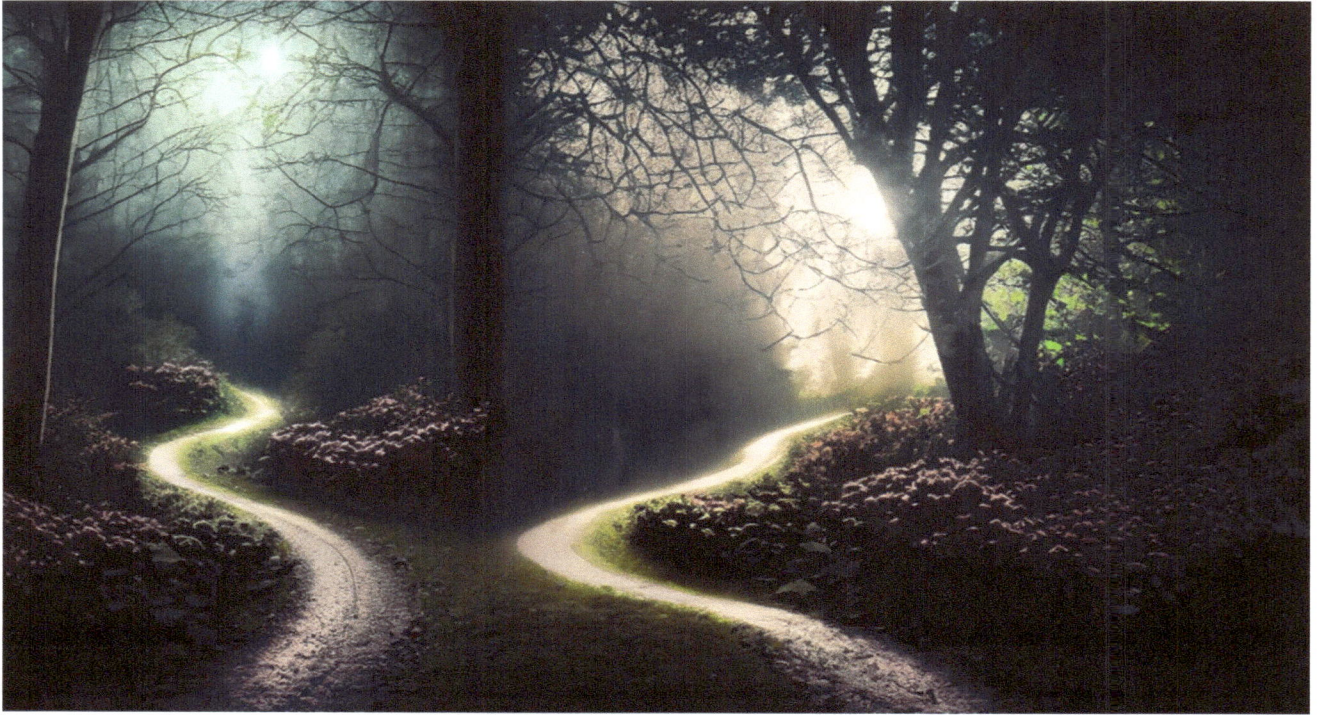

Dad leaned in, his voice dropping to a gentle tone. "Imagine there are two forces within each of us, Saumyaa, and Saharsha," he explained. "One force is like a bright light, guiding us towards goodness and compassion. These are the divine qualities, like honesty, kindness, and patience."

Saharsha's eyes widened with interest. "So, these good qualities are like sunshine, helping us grow and be happy?"

Dad chuckled. "Exactly, Saharsha! Just like sunshine helps a plant flourish, divine qualities help us become better people."

"And what about the other force, Dad?" Saumyaa inquired, her voice tinged with a hint of apprehension.

Dad nodded. "The other force is like a shadow, leading us towards negativity. These are the demonic qualities, such as greed, anger, and arrogance."

# THE STORIES WITHIN: LESSONS LEARNED IN THE LIGHT OF THE GITA

Dad, his voice taking on a warm, storytelling quality, leaned closer to Saumyaa and Saharsha. "The Bhagavad Gita," he began, "teaches us about our true selves, the Atman, and the impermanent nature of the material world. Today, we'll explore two stories that illustrate the importance of cultivating divine qualities (Satvic Gunas) and the pitfalls of succumbing to demonic qualities (Tamasic Gunas)."

## The Dog and the Bone: A Story About Wanting More

"Have you ever heard the story of Bruno, the dog who loved bones more than anything?" Dad asked with a twinkle in his eye.

Saumyaa and Saharsha shook their heads, eager to hear the tale.

Dad chuckled. "Well then, listen closely," he said, "because this story teaches a valuable lesson."

Bruno, a chubby Beagle with a tail that always wagged, lived happily with his loving owner, Sarah. Every afternoon, Sarah would take Bruno for a walk in the park where he'd play with all his might. One sunny day, as Bruno trotted along the familiar path, something caught his eye. It was a bone! The biggest, juiciest bone he'd ever seen!

Bruno couldn't resist. He snatched the bone right away, his tail wagging even faster. He imagined himself having a wonderful time chewing on his treasure. But remember, wanting more and more things can make us forget about the good things we already have.

Suddenly, Bruno crossed a narrow bridge over a babbling brook. He glanced down at the water's reflection and saw another dog – a sleek Doberman Pinscher – with an even bigger, juicier bone! Bruno's eyes widened in surprise. How unfair! He thought. That bone should be mine!

Without thinking, Bruno lunged towards the reflection, barking fiercely. He wanted to grab the bigger bone from the Doberman. But in his haste, Bruno forgot to be careful. He slipped on the narrow bridge and fell headfirst into the cool water below!

The bone he'd been so excited about slipped from his mouth and disappeared into the current. When Bruno finally climbed out, shivering and wet, the reflection and the bigger bone were gone. He searched everywhere for it, but it was nowhere to be found.

Bruno felt awful. In his foolish chase after something he didn't even have, he lost the delicious bone he already had.

## Lesson Learned: Be Happy with What You Have

Dad's voice softened as he finished the story. "This tale of Bruno, my dears, reminds us that wanting more and more things can make us unhappy. It can make us forget about the good things we already have. Remember, it's important to be happy with what you have and enjoy the present moment."

Saumyaa thought for a moment. "So, Dad, are we not supposed to want anything nice?" she asked.

Dad smiled warmly. "No, of course not, Saumyaa. It's okay to want nice things. But there's a difference between wanting something and getting greedy. We can enjoy good things in life, but we shouldn't let them control us."

## Queen Draupadi: Embracing Karma and Equanimity

"Now, let's explore a different story," Dad continued, his voice taking on a more contemplative tone. "This tale delves into the power of Karma and the importance of cultivating equanimity (Samata), a divine quality (Satvic Guna)."

He then narrated the captivating story of Queen Draupadi, a wise and beautiful ruler known for her strong spirit. In a previous life, Draupadi had performed a powerful penance, wishing for a husband with a specific set of qualities. This This action, according to the Bhagavad Gita, can be seen as fulfilling her Karma, the law of cause and effect. In her next life, her desires manifested, but not exactly as she had envisioned.

Dad explained the complexities of Draupadi's story, highlighting how her past actions (Karma) influenced her present circumstances. Despite the challenges of having five husbands with distinct personalities and strengths, Draupadi learned to accept her fate (Swadharma) with equanimity (Samata), a central theme in the Bhagavad Gita.

She focused on the positive qualities of each husband – Yudhisthira's righteousness, Bhima's immense strength, Arjuna's unmatched archery skills, Nakula's handsomeness, and Sahadeva's wisdom. This exemplifies the Bhagavad Gita's message of seeking the good in all situations.

She also learned to navigate their shortcomings with patience and understanding (Sattvic qualities). This demonstrates performing one's duty (Dharma) within the family unit, fostering a sense of unity and love.

Lesson Learned: The Fruits of Equanimity

"The story of Queen Draupadi," Dad explained, his voice filled with wisdom, "teaches us valuable lessons about *Karma, Dharma, and Samata* (equanimity), as illuminated by the Bhagavad Gita. We are all bound by our past actions, but we have the power to choose how we respond to our present circumstances. By cultivating equanimity we can accept what life throws our way, focusing on the positive aspects and performing our duties with a calm and composed mind."

"So, even if things don't go exactly as planned, we should stay calm and make the best of it?" Saharsha inquired, his brow furrowed in thought.

Dad nodded. "Precisely, Saharsha. The Bhagavad Gita teaches us that true happiness lies not in controlling the external world, but in mastering our inner world. By developing equanimity, we can navigate life's challenges with grace and resilience, building meaningful relationships and fulfilling our purpose."

By incorporating these revisions, the stories directly reference the Bhagavad Gita's teachings, providing a deeper connection between the narrative and the scripture. The revised passages also use terminology from the Bhagavad Gita, such as Dharma, Karma, and Samata, enriching the reader's understanding of these concepts.

## The Path Forward: Cultivating Goodness with the Bhagavad Gita as Our Guide

Saharsha pondered this for a moment. "So, everyone has both good and bad qualities, like the Pandavas in the Mahabharata?" he queried, referencing the epic Dad had mentioned earlier.

Dad nodded. "That's right, Saharsha. The Bhagavad Gita teaches us that we all contain both divine (Sattvic) and demonic (Tamasic) qualities. Recognizing these qualities within ourselves and striving to cultivate the divine ones, like those exemplified by the Pandavas in their righteous pursuit of Dharma, is what truly matters."

Saumyaa, ever the thoughtful one, chimed in, "Thank you for explaining, Dad. It seems like a lot of work to stay on the right path with so many temptations around us, just like Arjuna facing his own kin on the battlefield."

Dad acknowledged her concern. "You're right, Saumyaa," he said. "Staying true to our good qualities requires discipline and a strong moral compass. The Bhagavad Gita emphasizes the importance of fulfilling our Dharma (duty) with a sense of detachment (Vairagya). Surrounding ourselves with positive influences, practicing self-control (Indriya Nigraha), and reflecting on our actions (Svadhyaya) are all vital tools in this journey."

## Embracing Imperfections: Growth and Redemption on the Path of the Gita

"But what if we make mistakes, Dad?" Saharsha asked, a hint of worry in his voice. "Does that mean we're bad, like the Kauravas who chose the path of Adharma (unrighteousness)?"

Dad's smile remained warm. "Not at all, Saharsha," he reassured him. "The Bhagavad Gita reminds us that everyone makes mistakes. The important thing is to learn from them, seek forgiveness when needed (Kshama), and strive to do better next time. Every day is a new opportunity to grow and become the best version of ourselves, just like Arjuna overcame his doubts and fulfilled his Dharma."

## The Seeds of Transformation: Cultivating a Garden of Virtue

To solidify this message, Dad presented another story, perhaps one that highlights the importance of perseverance and overcoming challenges. "Let's hear the inspiring tale of..." Dad's voice took on a gentle, almost earthy quality as he began the tale of the farmer and the seeds.

"There once was a farmer named Raj, known throughout the land for his dedication to his craft," Dad began. "Each year, Raj meticulously prepared his fields, tilling the soil with care and ensuring it was rich with nutrients. He then carefully selected his seeds – plump, healthy kernels that promised bountiful harvests."

Raj, unlike some farmers who opted for quick-growing, low-yield crops, believed in quality over quantity. He planted seeds renowned for their deliciousness and resilience, knowing the extra effort would pay off in the long run.

"The day finally arrived for sowing," Dad continued. "Raj, with a weathered hand and a rhythmic stride, scattered the seeds across his fields. Some seeds landed on fertile patches of earth, basking in the warm sunshine. Others landed near sturdy rocks, their roots finding ways to burrow deeper and access the life-giving moisture below."

Unfortunately, not all the seeds found such ideal conditions. A few fell on hard, sun-baked ground, offering little hope for growth. Others landed amongst a flurry of weeds, their access to sunlight and nutrients threatened.

"Despite the uneven terrain," Dad explained, "Raj continued to care for his fields with unwavering dedication. He watered the thirsty seedlings, cleared away encroaching weeds, and protected them from hungry pests."

As weeks turned into months, a transformation unfolded. The seeds that fell on fertile ground sprouted with vigor, their leaves reaching for the sun. Even those nestled near rocks displayed an unexpected resilience, their roots pushing through cracks in search of sustenance.

However, the seeds on the hardened ground remained dormant, their journey ending before it even began. The seeds choked by weeds struggled for survival, their growth stunted by the competition.

"Harvest time arrived, and Raj's dedication bore fruit," Dad announced, a hint of pride in his voice. "The fields that had once held tiny seeds now boasted tall, healthy stalks laden with plump, delicious vegetables. The harvest was bountiful, a testament to Raj's patience and care."

## The Lesson of Perseverance

"This story, my dears," Dad concluded, his voice warm, "holds a valuable lesson. Just like the farmer's seeds, we all have the potential to grow and flourish. However, like the seeds that faced challenges, we too may encounter obstacles – moments of doubt, temptations to stray from the right path, or difficult circumstances. But just as Raj nurtured his seeds with unwavering care, we must cultivate perseverance and a commitment to our goals."

"So, even if things seem difficult, we should keep working hard?" Saharsha inquired, his brow furrowed in thought.

Dad nodded. "Exactly, Saharsha. Remember, the journey towards inner light requires dedication, just like Raj's dedication to his crops. With perseverance and a focus on cultivating good qualities, we can overcome challenges and blossom into the best versions of ourselves."

He then narrated the story, highlighting how the farmer's dedication, despite challenges, led to bountiful crops. "Just like the farmer cultivates his land, we can cultivate our inner garden," Dad concluded. "By planting seeds of kindness (Maitri), compassion (Karuna), and generosity (Dana), as emphasized in the Bhagavad Gita, we create a world of goodness, enriching not only ourselves but everyone around us."

## The Journey Continues: A World Transformed by the Light of the Gita

Saumyaa and Saharsha sat in thoughtful silence, reflecting on the stories and Dad's words. "Thank you, Dad," Saumyaa finally spoke, her voice filled with gratitude. "These stories and the lessons from the Bhagavad Gita have shown us how important it is to choose the path of light."

Dad squeezed their shoulders gently. "You're welcome, my dears," he replied. "Remember, the journey towards inner light, guided by the wisdom of the Bhagavad Gita, continues throughout life. As you grow and learn, you'll encounter new challenges and opportunities to strengthen your divine qualities. By staying committed to living with integrity and compassion, you'll not only illuminate your own path but also inspire others to do the same."

## CHAPTER SUMMARY: DIVINE QUALITIES VS DEMONIC QUALITIES

This chapter explores the reasons behind people's choices and actions. Dad explains that everyone has a mix of good (divine) and bad (demonic) qualities that influence how we behave.

- **Divine Qualities:** These are positive qualities like honesty, kindness, and forgiveness. They lead to good behavior and a happy life.

- **Demonic Qualities:** These are negative qualities like lying, greed, and anger. They can lead us down the wrong path and create problems.

The chapter emphasizes the importance of developing good habits and letting go of bad ones. It uses stories like "The Dog and the Bone" and "Queen Draupadi" to illustrate the consequences of bad choices and the importance of accepting both good and bad qualities in ourselves and others.

While Dad acknowledges the difficulty of staying on the right path, he offers guidance:

- **Surrounding ourselves with positive influences**: Spending time with good people can inspire us to be better.

- **Self-discipline**: Controlling our impulses and making good choices, even when it's hard.

- **Reflection**: Taking time to think about our actions and how they affect ourselves and others.

Finally, the chapter uses the story of "The Farmer and the Seeds" to show that even with challenges, we can cultivate our inner garden of good qualities. The chapter concludes with an inspiring message: each person has the power to spread kindness and compassion, making the world a better place.

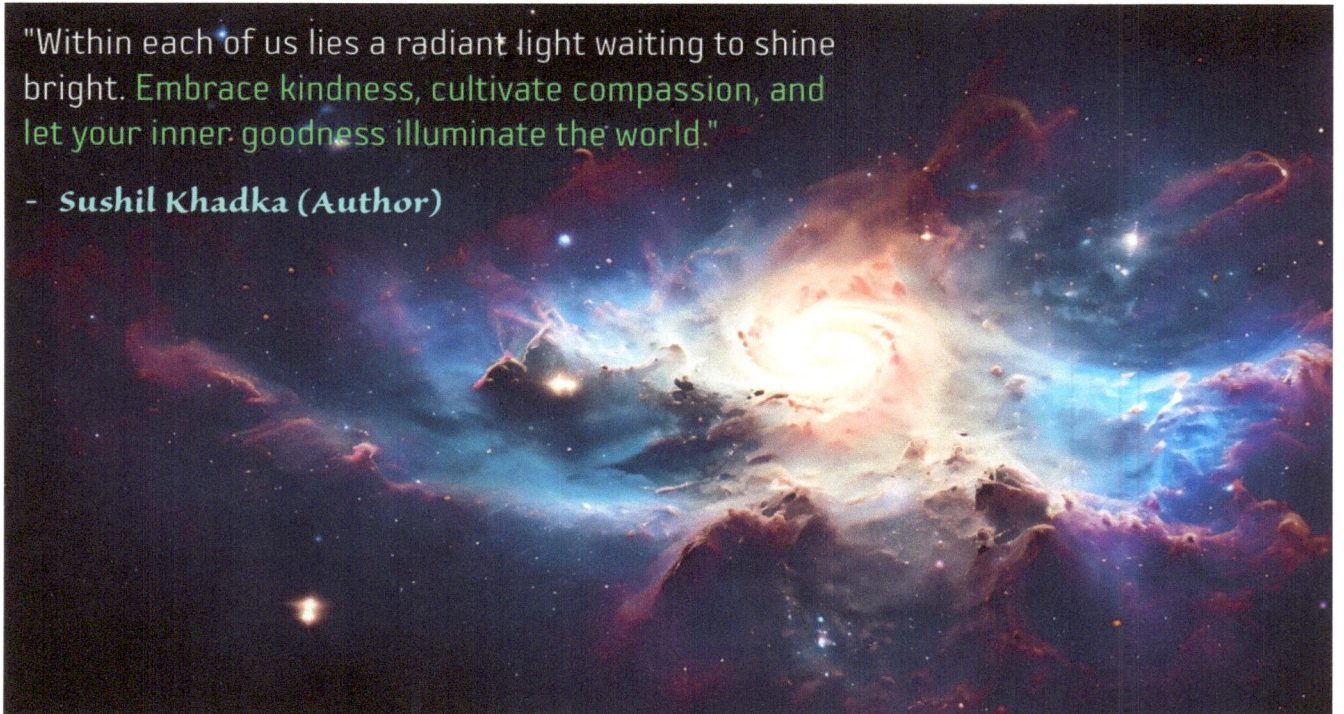

"Within each of us lies a radiant light waiting to shine bright. Embrace kindness, cultivate compassion, and let your inner goodness illuminate the world."

- Sushil Khadka (Author)

# Chapter 17: Guiding Lights: Nourishing Body, Mind, and Soul

"

## *Secrets of the Inner Playground*

*Enter a realm where the ordinary becomes extraordinary, where the mundane transforms into mystery. Join Saumyaa and Saharsha as they unlock the hidden truths of body, mind, and soul in Chapter 17: Guiding Lights: Nourishing Body, Mind, and Soul. Prepare for a mind-bending journey through the Sunshine Playground, the Bouncy Castle Playground, and the Quiet Cave. Unravel perplexing tales of balance and discovery, where every twist reveals a new puzzle piece in the enigmatic tapestry of life. Dare to embark on this tantalizing adventure, where mysteries await around every corner.*

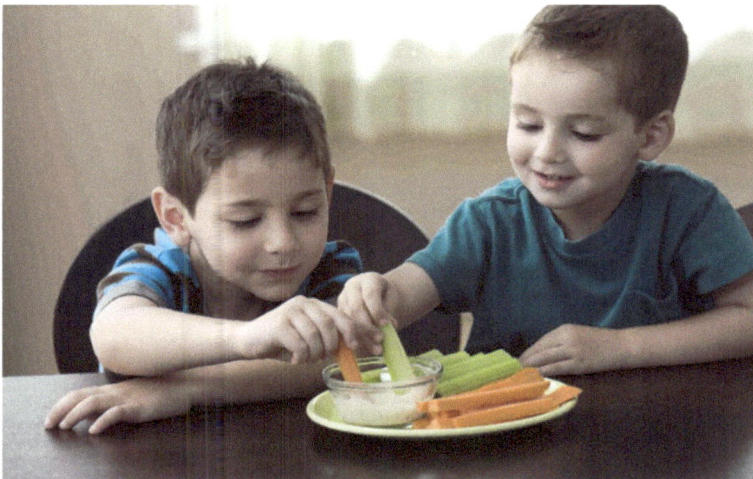

The warm afternoon sun peeked through the window, painting golden squares on the living room rug.

Saumyaa, always curious, tilted her head like a puppy listening for a treat. "Dad," she asked, "how do we make good choices in life, even about things like what we eat?"

Dad chuckled, his eyes crinkling at the corners. "That's a great question, Saumyaa. Imagine there are three kinds of food in the world, like three different playgrounds."

Saharsha's eyes gleamed with interest. "Playgrounds? Cool!"

Dad smiled. "The first playground is Sattva Playground. It's full of sunshine and healthy snacks like fruits and veggies. Kids who play there feel energized but calm, ready to learn and be kind."

"Like a jungle gym with slides and swings, but with healthy snacks instead of cookies?" Saumyaa clarified.

Dad laughed. "Exactly! Now, Rajas Playground is more like a giant bouncy castle. It's super fun, with spicy foods and sugary treats that give you a burst of energy. But sometimes, too much bouncing can make you feel jittery or tired."

Saharsha scrunched his nose. "Like having too much cake at a birthday party?"

"Perfect example!" Dad agreed. "The last playground is Tamas Playground. It's kind of dark and quiet, with heavy foods that make you sluggish, like if you only ate French fries all day."

Saumyaa wrinkled her nose. "Sounds boring!"

Dad nodded. "Exactly. So, the key is to balance your time between all the playgrounds. Have fun on the bouncy castle (Rajas) sometimes, but mostly play in the sunshine (Sattva) with healthy snacks. And avoid spending too much time in the dark playground (Tamas)."

"So, eating healthy isn't just about not getting sick, it's about having the most fun on the sunshine playground?" Saumyaa concluded.

Dad beamed. "Absolutely, Saumyaa! When you eat good food, you feel good and have the energy to be kind and helpful to others."

Inspired by this conversation, Saharsha piped up, "Dad, you mentioned helping others earlier. How can we really make a difference?"

"Helping others," Dad explained, "is like playing a superhero game. You don't need fancy gadgets, just a kind heart. Remember the story of the little ant who helped a lost baby bird?"

Saumyaa's eyes widened. "A tiny ant helping a bird? How?"

"The ant," Dad continued, "carried a tiny piece of bread to the bird's nest, even though it seemed like a small thing. But that small act of kindness helped the baby bird survive!"

Saharsha grinned. "So even small things can make a big difference?"

Dad nodded. "Exactly! You can be a superhero by helping a neighbor carry grocery, volunteering at an animal shelter, or simply sharing your toys with a friend."

A thoughtful silence fell upon them.

"Dad," Saharsha spoke hesitantly, "you said something about faith before. What's that?"

Dad's voice softened. "Faith is like having a special compass inside you that helps you choose the right path. It's about believing in yourself, even when things are tough. Like when a brave knight sets out on a quest, he has faith that he can overcome any obstacle."

Saumyaa's eyes sparkled. "So, faith helps us be strong and courageous?"

Dad smiled. "Yes, Saumyaa! By believing in good things and doing good deeds, our faith grows stronger, like a seed that blossoms into a beautiful flower."

As their conversation flowed like a gentle stream, each question a stepping stone, the family felt a sense of wonder about the world around them. Stories sparked their imaginations, and with each new concept, they learned valuable lessons about making good choices, helping others, and believing in themselves.

As the conversation deepened, Saumyaa, ever the inquisitive one, furrowed her brow. "But Dad," she interjected, "what if I accidentally end up in the Tamas Playground too much? Like if I have a bad day and just want to eat ice cream and watch cartoons all day?"

Dad chuckled warmly. "That happens to everyone sometimes, Saumyaa. Nobody's perfect! The important thing is to recognize when you've strayed a bit too far and gently guide yourself back to the sunshine. Maybe after that ice cream and cartoon marathon, you can take a walk outside, get some fresh air, and feel that Sattva energy come back."

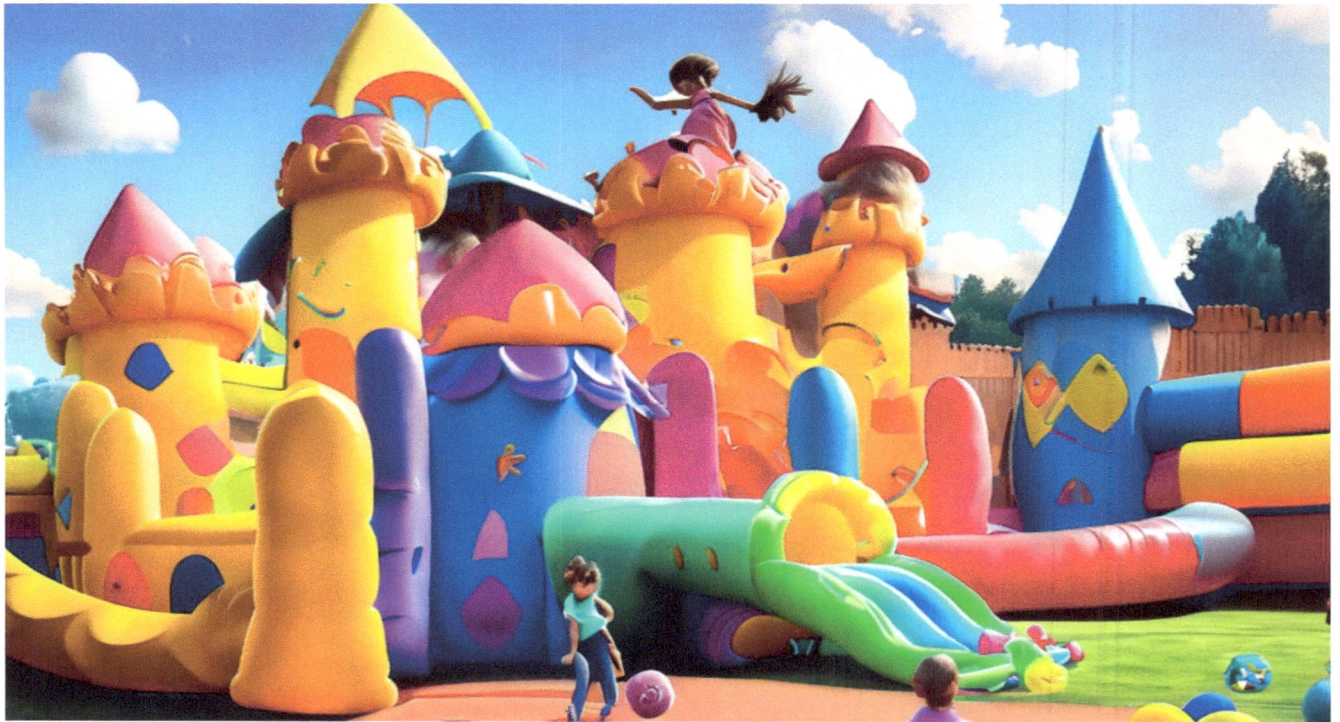

Saharsha, now lost in thought, chimed in, "So, these playgrounds represent how we feel and act too, right? Like if I'm always super energetic and bouncing off the walls, that's Rajas?"

Dad's eyes lit up. "Exactly, Saharsha! It's all connected. When you're feeling restless or argumentative, that might be a sign of too much Rajas energy. Maybe taking some deep breaths or doing some calming yoga poses can help you find your center again."

The conversation sparked a fire of curiosity in Saumyaa. Her eyes, usually sparkling with mischief, now held a deep earnestness. "Dad," she asked, her voice hushed with a newfound respect for the power of faith, "can you tell us a story about someone who used their faith to overcome a challenge?"

Dad's smile widened, his eyes crinkling at the corners as he surveyed his enthralled children. A lifetime of stories seemed to dance behind his eyelids. "Ah," he began, his voice taking on a gentle, almost rhythmic quality, "there are many such tales woven into the fabric of time, Saumyaa. Each one a testament to the strength of the human spirit."

He paused for a moment, letting the anticipation build. "Once upon a time," he continued, his voice weaving a spell, "in a village nestled amidst rolling hills, lived a young girl named Priya. Unlike other children who reveled in the playful dance of fireflies at dusk, Priya dreaded the approach of night. As the sun dipped below the horizon, shadows stretched across her room, morphing into monstrous shapes in her imagination. Fear, cold and constricting, would grip her heart, whispering tales of lurking dangers."

Saharsha, who had been fidgeting moments ago, was now completely still, captivated by the story. He leaned forward, his brow furrowed in concern for the young Priya.

Dad continued, his voice a soothing balm. "But Priya, even in the face of her fear, possessed a flicker of faith. It was a tiny flame, nurtured by the stories her grandmother used to tell her – stories of brave heroes and unwavering spirits. Every night, as the shadows began their dance, Priya would remember those tales and a small, determined voice would rise within her."

He gestured towards his chest, mimicking the rise of courage. "Taking a deep breath, Priya would sing a special song her grandmother had taught her. It was a simple melody, filled with words of hope and bravery. As the song filled the room, the shadows seemed to lose their menacing forms. With each note, Priya felt a sliver of her fear melt away, replaced by a newfound sense of calm."

Dad's voice softened to a whisper. "It wasn't an overnight victory. There were nights when the shadows seemed more terrifying than ever. But Priya never gave up on her faith or her song. Slowly, bit by bit, the fear lost its grip on her. The shadows remained, but they no longer held the power to control her."

As the sun dipped below the horizon, casting warm orange and purple hues across the room, a comfortable silence settled. The family felt a deep sense of connection, their hearts brimming with a newfound understanding.

Each question, like a stepping stone, had led them on a path of self-discovery. Saumyaa's eyes sparkled with a newfound determination to make good choices, while Saharsha, his usual restlessness replaced by a newfound calm, seemed to ponder the power of faith. With hearts full of wonder and a renewed sense of purpose, they knew their journey of learning had just begun.

Perhaps tomorrow, Dad would share another story, or maybe they'd put their newfound knowledge to the test by planning healthy snacks for the next day's adventure. The possibilities, like the universe itself, stretched before them, vast and full of wonder.

## CHAPTER SUMMARY: GUIDING LIGHTS: NOURISHING BODY, MIND, AND SOUL

This chapter explores the interconnectedness of physical health, mental well-being, and spiritual growth, using engaging stories and relatable metaphors for children.

### The Three Guiding Lights:

The chapter introduces three guiding lights that illuminate our path:

- **Nourishing the Body (Sattva):** Explained through the Sunshine Playground. Here, children imagine a place filled with healthy foods like fruits and vegetables, sunshine, and activities that promote calmness and good health. This highlights healthy choices as fuel for a strong body and clear mind.

- **Engaging the Mind (Rajas):** Represented by the Bouncy Castle Playground. This playground symbolizes activities that bring excitement and energy. It's okay to have fun here, but too much bouncing (too much Rajas energy) can lead to restlessness. Spicy foods and sugary treats are examples of things that can have a Rajasic effect.

- **Finding Inner Peace (Tamas):** Envisioned as the Quiet Cave. While not inherently bad, spending too much time here can lead to sluggishness and a lack of motivation. Deep-fried foods and excessive screen time are examples of Tamasic influences.

## The Importance of Balance:

The chapter emphasizes the importance of finding balance between these three guiding lights. We should spend most of our time in the Sunshine Playground, enjoying healthy activities and foods that promote well-being. Brief visits to the Bouncy Castle Playground are okay for bursts of excitement, and the Quiet Cave can be a place for relaxation, but not for too long.

## Kindness and Faith: The Extra Twinkle:

Going beyond physical well-being, the chapter highlights the importance of kindness and faith. Stories like the one about the little ant helping a baby bird illustrate the power of small acts of charity. Faith is explained as a special light within us, like a compass that helps us choose the right path and overcome challenges. The story of Priya conquering her fear of the dark through faith in a song exemplifies this concept.

# Chapter 18: Adventures in Selflessness

"

## *Selflessness Unveiled: Journeys of Compassion*

*As the afternoon sun dips, a family delves into a world of selflessness, pondering its mysteries with childlike curiosity. Join Saharsha, Saumyaa, and Dad on a quest to unravel the enigma of ego, explore the joy of service, and embark on adventures in selflessness. Through captivating tales of ancient wisdom and heartfelt discussions, discover how even the smallest acts of kindness can illuminate the path to true happiness. Get ready to journey beyond the boundaries of self and into a realm, where compassion reigns supreme. Adventures in Selflessness awaits, beckoning you to explore, reflect, and grow.*

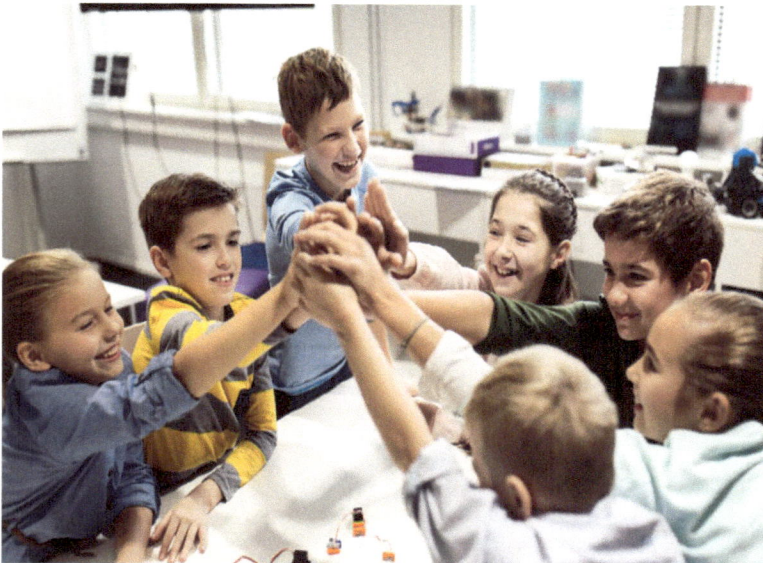

The afternoon sun dipped lower in the sky, casting long shadows across the living room rug. Saharsha, brow furrowed in concentration, finally broke the comfortable silence. "Dad," he said, his voice laced with confusion, "this whole idea of not caring about getting anything back for helping others seems weird. Can you explain it in a way that makes sense to kids like us?"

Dad chuckled warmly, his eyes crinkling at the corners. "Absolutely, Saharsha. It's not about becoming a hermit and living alone! It's more about letting go of selfishness, like when you only want to play with a toy if it's yours and refuse to share."

Saumyaa, ever the curious one, scrunched up her nose. "Dad, what exactly is this 'ego' you keep talking about? Is it like a tiny voice bossing us around inside our heads?"

Dad chuckled. "That's a great way to think about it, Saumyaa! Imagine you have a little chatterbox inside your head. This voice reminds you of all the cool things you can do, how good you are at drawing or playing soccer, and maybe even brags a little sometimes. That's your ego!"

Saharsha piped in, "So, it's like our inner cheerleader?"

Dad smiled. ' Exactly, Saharsha! Having an ego isn't a bad thing. It can give you a confidence boost and make you feel proud of your accomplishments. But sometimes, that little cheerleader can get a bit carried away."

Saumyaa giggled. "Like when it whispers, 'I'm the best, and everyone else should listen to me'?'

Dad winked. 'Spot on, Saumyaa! That's when it's important to remember that everyone has an ego, just like you. We all have things we're good at and things we need to work on. The key is to listen to your ego sometimes, but not all the time."

Our ego can be a tricky character, whispering in our ears that we're the most important and deserve all the credit. But the truth is, we're all part of something much bigger than ourselves. Take the story of Siddhartha Gautama, the Buddha himself."

Saharsha's eyes widened. "The Buddha? But wasn't he a prince who left his palace and all his riches?"

Dad smiled. "Indeed, Saharsha. Siddhartha lived a sheltered life, unaware of the suffering in the world. Yet, a deep yearning for truth and understanding drove him to leave his palace. He journeyed far and wide, seeking answers to life's mysteries. Through his experiences and meditations, he realized true happiness doesn't come from material possessions or fleeting pleasures."

Saumyaa pondered this for a moment. "So, the Buddha found happiness by giving up everything?"

Dad shook his head gently. "Not quite, Saumyaa. He found happiness by letting go of his attachment to things. He realized that true joy comes from within, from a place of peace and compassion. He then dedicated his life to teaching others how to find this inner peace and freedom from suffering."

A thoughtful silence descended upon them.

Saharsha finally spoke, his voice laced with curiosity. "But Dad, what about jobs and responsibilities? How can we be selfless if we have things to do?"

Dad's smile widened. "Think of your work as an opportunity for service, Saharsha. Imagine Queen Jhansi of India, a courageous leader who fought for her people's freedom. She used her position not for personal gain, but to protect those in need."

Saumyaa's eyes sparkled with understanding. "So, it's not about the job itself, but the intention behind it?"

Dad beamed. "Precisely, Saumyaa! Even the smallest tasks, done with kindness and dedication, can be acts of service. Remember the story of Florence Nightingale, the famous nurse who revolutionized patient care? She wasn't motivated by wealth or fame, but by a deep compassion for the sick and injured."

Saharsha, ever the pragmatist, chimed in again. "But Dad, sometimes it's hard to be selfless, especially when everyone else seems to be focused on themselves."

Dad placed a hand on Saharsha's shoulder, his voice filled with reassurance. "It's true, Saharsha. It takes courage and effort to choose selflessness. But remember, even small acts of kindness can ripple outward, inspiring others to do the same. Take the story of the little boy who offered his single lunch to a hungry stranger. His simple act of compassion sparked a chain reaction of generosity."

Saumyaa, a flicker of determination in her eyes, concluded the conversation. "So, adventures in selflessness are all about letting go of ego, serving others, and making the world a better place, even in small ways?"

Dad's face lit up with pride. "Absolutely, Saumyaa! Every time you choose kindness over selfishness, you embark on an incredible adventure that benefits not only others but also yourself. Remember, within each of us lies the potential for great compassion and selflessness. By following the path of the *Buddha, Queen Jhansi, Florence Nightingale,* or even the little boy with his lunch, we can all embark on these extraordinary adventures in selflessness."

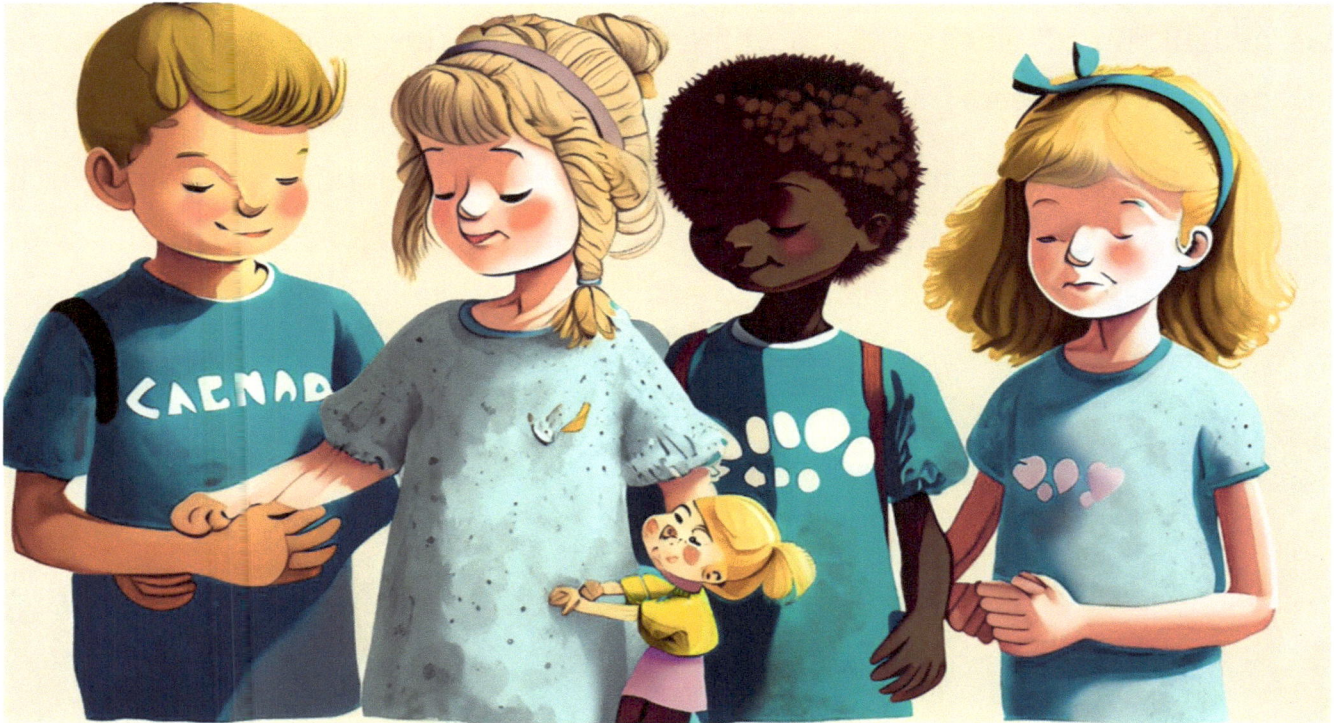

As the sun dipped below the horizon, casting long shadows across the room, the family felt a deep sense of connection and purpose. They understood that true happiness lay not in acquiring things, but in letting go of ego and serving others. Their journey of learning had just begun, filled with the promise of exciting adventures in selflessness.

The next day, the spirit of exploration sparked by the conversation lingered.

Saharsha: Dad, you mentioned the Buddha found happiness through meditation. Can we try that too?

Dad: Absolutely, Saharsha! Meditation is a practice of quieting your mind and focusing your attention. Even a few minutes a day can help you feel calmer and more centered. There are many simple techniques, like focusing on your breath, that we can try together.

Saumyaa: Can we meditate on becoming more selfless?

Dad: That's a wonderful idea, Saumyaa! As you focus on your breath, imagine sending out feelings of kindness and compassion to everyone around you. Picture a warm light spreading outwards, touching the people you love, your classmates, even strangers on the street.

Activity: Dad guided them through a simple breathing meditation, focusing on each inhale and exhale. They then visualized sending out waves of kindness, starting with their family and gradually expanding to encompass the whole world.

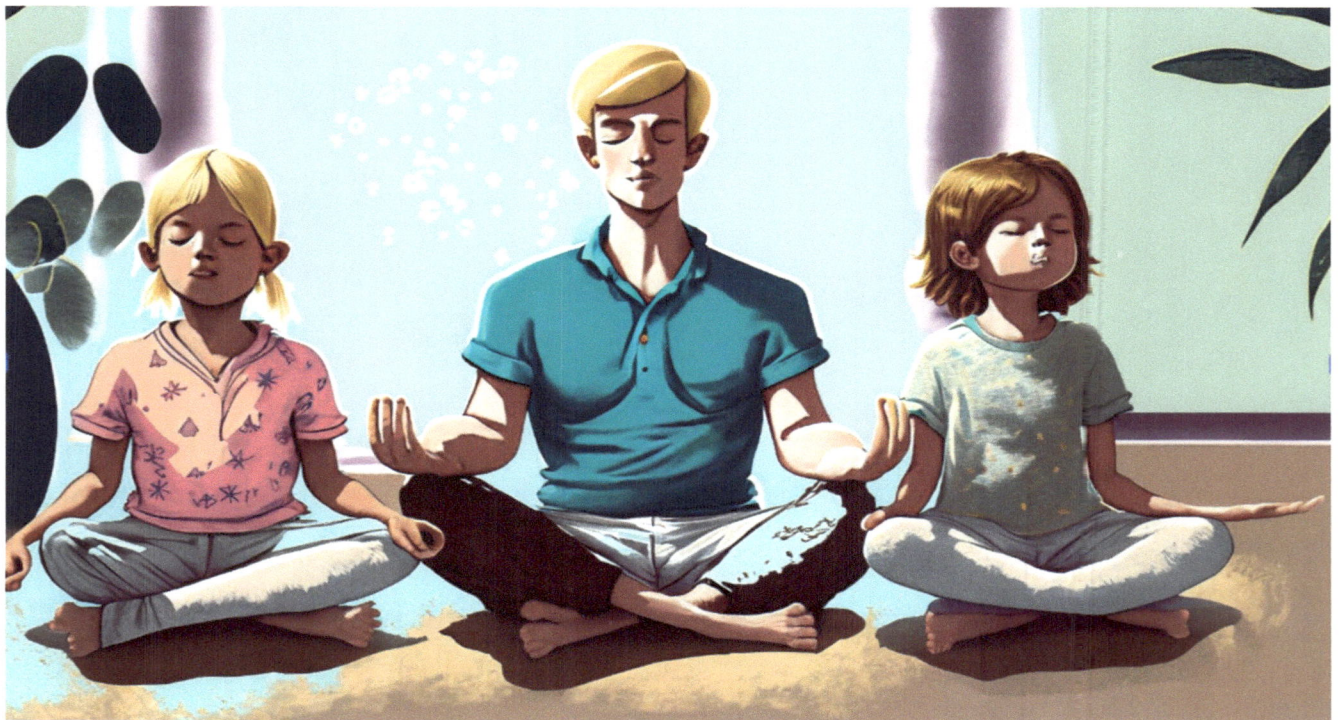

Saharsha: Wow, Dad! I felt a warm glow inside when I thought about helping others.

Saumyaa: Me too! It felt good.

Dad: That's the power of meditation, Saumyaa. When we cultivate compassion within ourselves, it becomes easier to act selflessly in the real world.

Putting it into Practice: Inspired by their meditation, the family brainstormed ways to translate their newfound awareness into action.

Saharsha: Maybe we can volunteer at the animal shelter on weekends?

Saumyaa: Yes! And we can sort out our old toys and donate them to kids who don't have many.

Dad: Those are fantastic ideas! Every act of kindness, no matter how small, makes a difference.

Challenges and Growth: As they embarked on their adventures in selflessness, the family encountered challenges.

Saharsha: Dad, I wanted to share my new game with a friend today, but he wasn't interested in playing the same thing.

Dad: It can be frustrating when your efforts aren't reciprocated, Saharsha. But remember, selflessness isn't about getting something back. It's about offering kindness without expecting anything in return. Maybe next time, you can suggest playing something he enjoys.

Saumyaa: What if some people seem grumpy or don't appreciate our help?

Dad: That's a good question, Saumyaa. Some people may be closed off to kindness at first. But by continuing to offer our help with a genuine smile, we can slowly break down those barriers. It's like watering a plant – it may not bloom overnight, but with patience and care, it will eventually blossom.

Continuing the Journey: Through their challenges and triumphs, the family discovered the joy of giving back and the interconnectedness of all beings. They learned that adventures in selflessness weren't just one-time events, but a lifelong journey of growth and compassion.

Final Thoughts: As the chapter drew to a close, the family reflected on their newfound understanding. They realized that true happiness came not from material possessions or fleeting pleasures, but from a life filled with service, kindness, and a sense of being part of something bigger than themselves. Their adventures in selflessness had just begun, and they were eager to see where the path would lead them next.

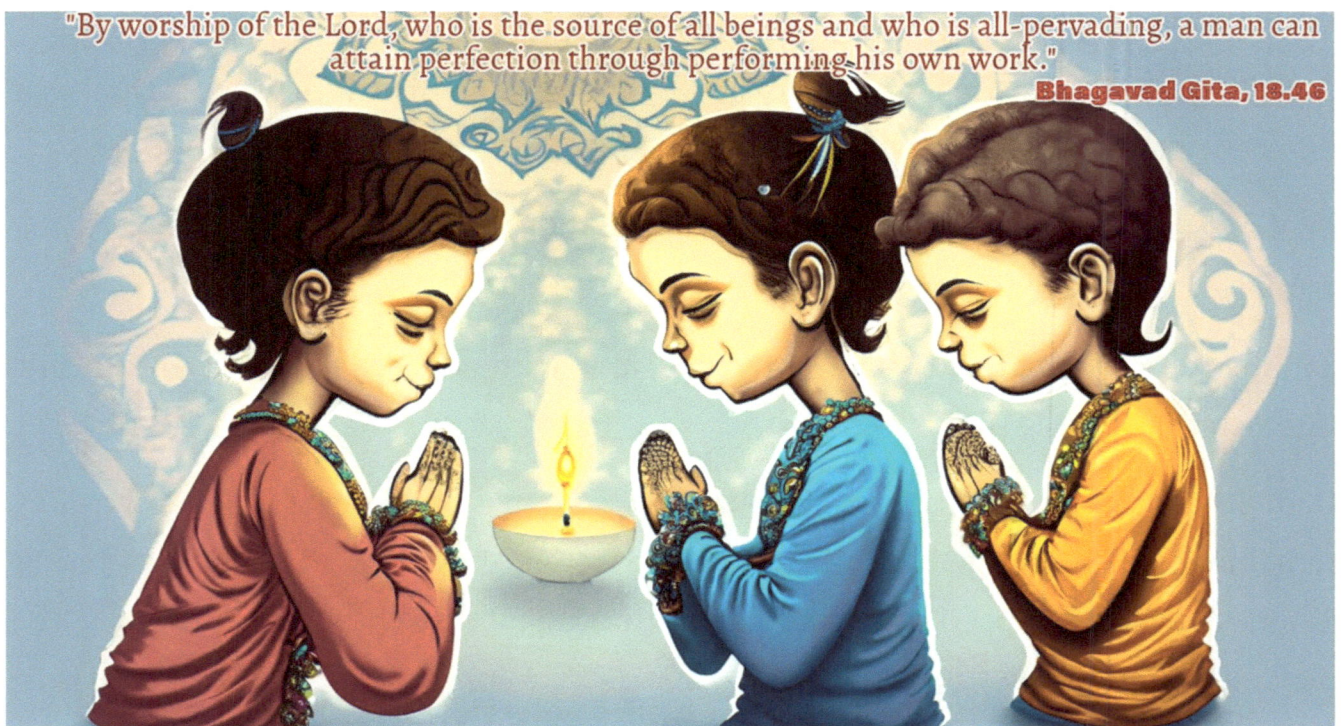

"By worship of the Lord, who is the source of all beings and who is all-pervading, a man can attain perfection through performing his own work."

Bhagavad Gita, 18.46

## CHAPTER SUMMARY: ADVENTURES IN SELFLESSNESS

This chapter explores the concept of selflessness and how it can lead to a happier and more fulfilling life. It uses stories from history and relatable activities to engage children.

## Letting Go of Ego:

- The chapter begins by explaining that selflessness isn't about abandoning everything, but about letting go of a self-centered attitude.

- The story of Siddhartha Gautama, the Buddha, is used as an example of someone who found happiness by letting go of attachment to material possessions.

## Service as a Source of Happiness:

- The concept of service is introduced through the story of Queen Jhansi, who used her power to protect others.

- Florence Nightingale's dedication to patient care exemplifies how even small acts done with kindness can be significant.

## Making a Difference:

- The importance of even small acts of kindness is emphasized through the story of a boy who shared his lunch with a stranger.

- Children are encouraged to reflect on how they can be selfless in their daily lives.

- A guided meditation exercise helps children experience the feeling of compassion.

## Putting Kindness into Action:

- The chapter outlines practical ways for children to be selfless, such as volunteering or donating toys.

## Challenges and Growth:

- The chapter acknowledges that being selfless isn't always easy.

- It explores how to deal with situations where kindness isn't reciprocated or appreciated.

- The importance of patience and perseverance in cultivating compassion is emphasized.

## Lifelong Journey:

- The chapter concludes with the idea that selflessness is a lifelong journey of growth and learning.

- Children are left with a sense of purpose and the motivation to continue their adventures in selflessness.

## Overall Message:

This chapter encourages children to develop compassion and selflessness as a way to find true happiness and contribute to a better world. It emphasizes the importance of service, kindness, and the interconnectedness of all beings.

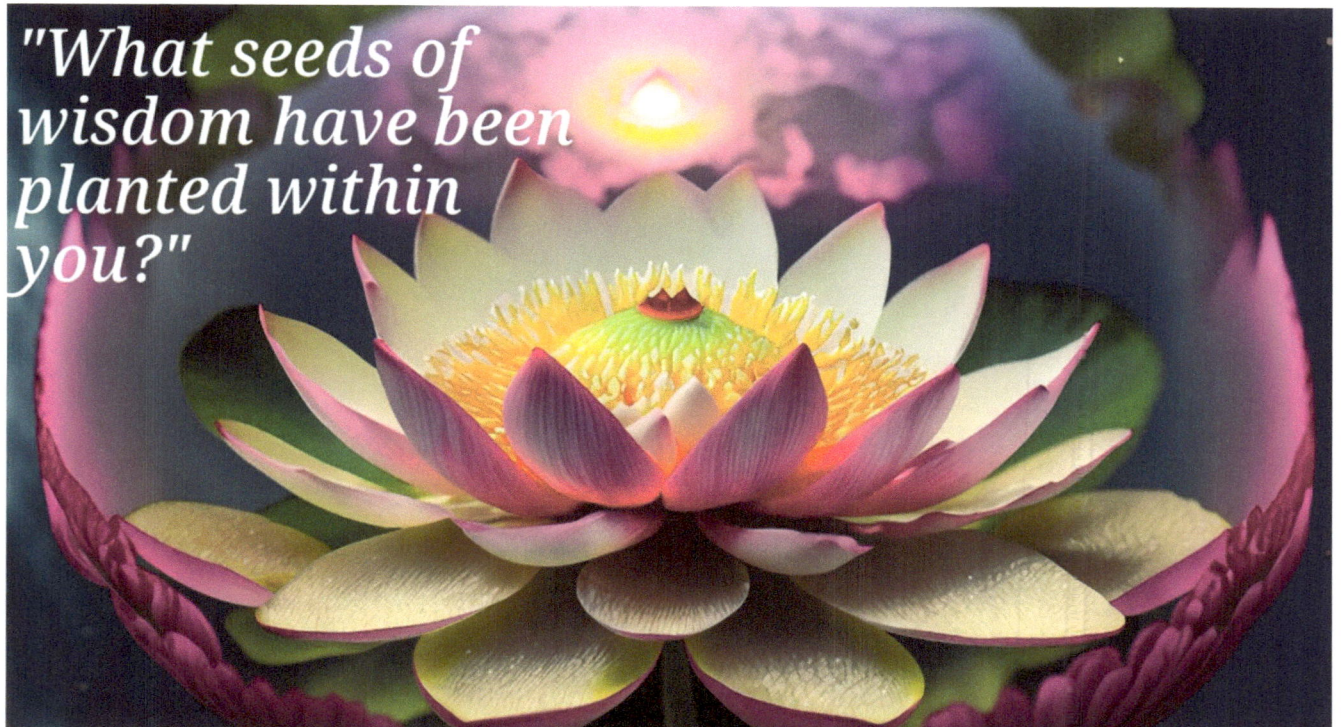

"What seeds of wisdom have been planted within you?"

# THE BHAGAVAD GITA WISDOM FOR YOUNG MINDS

Join Saharsha and Saumyaa on a heartwarming adventure as they unlock the wisdom of the Bhagavad Gita!

This captivating guidebook makes ancient wisdom accessible for young minds, fostering curiosity, self-discovery, and a connection with the Divine.

---

## Synopsis:

### Crack the Code: Bhagavad Gita for Young Minds

Forget dusty texts! This interactive adventure unlocks the Bhagavad Gita's wisdom for YOU.
Unveil secrets with a captivating story, then **EMBARK** on a **QUEST!**

Face challenges, find your path, and be the hero of your own story.

### The Bhagavad Gita: Wisdom for Today's Young Minds.

---

## SUSHIL KHADKA

Sushil Khadka is a dedicated explorer of both earthly and cosmic realms. For over 22 years, he has delved into mystic sciences like Vedic Astrology, Vaastu Shastra, Feng Shui, Tantra, and Tarot reading.

Sushil Khadka's journey harmoniously blends the material and the metaphysical, weaving a tapestry of enlightenment.

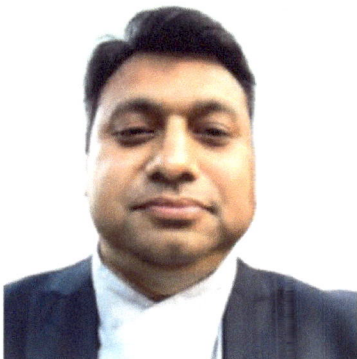